MCQs and Revision Aid
Medicine

MCQs and Revision Aid in Occupational Medicine

Ken Addley MB, MRCGP, MICGP, MFOM
Director, Occupational Health Service, Northern Ireland Civil Service, Belfast

With a Foreword by W. A. Eakins CBE, FFOM, DL

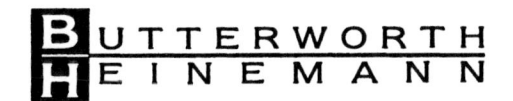

BUTTERWORTH
HEINEMANN

Butterworth-Heinemann Ltd
Linacre House, Jordan Hill, Oxford OX2 8DP

A member of the Reed Elsevier plc group

OXFORD LONDON BOSTON
MUNICH NEW DELHI SINGAPORE SYDNEY
TOKYO TORONTO WELLINGTON

First published 1995

© Butterworth-Heinemann Ltd 1995

All rights reserved. No part of this publication
may be reproduced in any material form (including
photocopying or storing in any medium by electronic
means and whether or not transiently or incidentally
to some other use of this publication) without the
written permission of the copyright holder except
in accordance with the provisions of the Copyright,
Designs and Patents Act 1988 or under the terms of a
licence issued by the Copyright Licensing Agency Ltd,
90 Tottenham Court Road, London, England W1P 9HE.
Applications for the copyright holder's written permission
to reproduce any part of this publication should be addressed
to the publishers

British Library Cataloguing in Publication Data
A catalogue record for this book is available from the British Library.

ISBN 0 7506 2394 2

Library of Congress Cataloguing in Publication Data
A catalogue record for this book is available from the Library of Congress.

Typeset by P&R Typesetters Ltd, Salisbury, Wilts

Contents

Foreword	vii
Preface	ix
Introduction	1
History and development of occupational medicine	3
Legal issues	5
Occupational hygiene	15
Physical hazards	21
Respiratory disorders	35
Occupational dermatoses	41
Occupational cancers	47
Ergonomics	51
Microbiological hazards	55
Mental health	63
Medical examinations	67
General toxicology	79
Epidemiology and statistics	97
Appendix A Common causes of occupational asthma	105
Appendix B Common causes of occupational dermatitis	106
Appendix C Occupations associated with contact dermatitis	107
Appendix D Occupational exposure limits	108
Further reading	112
Useful addresses	113

Foreword

Occupational medicine has a very wide clinical base and no one occupational physician's duties are likely to make him/her familiar with all the many toxic or physical hazards faced by workforces throughout industry today.

This comprehensive revision aid, in MCQ form, will be of benefit to two groups of people. Firstly, the post graduate student, be they general practitioners or full time in the speciality, who will find it useful as a quick reminder of the spectrum of knowledge required for AFOM/Diploma London and LFOM/MFOM Dublin. Secondly, it will act as a refresher and reminder for those of us who have been practising for some years in one particular aspect of the speciality, perhaps in isolation.

The author is to be congratulated on a valuable revision tool.

W. A. Eakins CBE, FFOM, DL
Belfast

Preface

The stimulus for this book came from my experience of sitting postgraduate examinations in the speciality and the absence of a quick revision aid which I would have found most helpful in my preparations. *MCQs and Revision Aid in Occupational Medicine* is therefore intended to meet the need of candidates preparing for examinations and will also be of benefit to those mature students who wish to test the depth of their current knowledge.

Occupational medicine has become increasingly important not least because of the plethora of health and safety legislation in the early 1990s. As a consequence many professionals have been attracted to it who are keen to obtain a qualification in the speciality. The extent of involvement, e.g. sessional, part-time or full-time, usually dictates the level of academic attainment. This text is aimed primarily at those medical practitioners studying for the Associateship of the Royal College of Physicians (London), the Licentiate and Membership of the Royal College of Physicians of Ireland, and general practitioners who intend sitting the Diploma examination organized by the Faculty of Occupational Medicine, Royal College of Physicians (London).

In addition, because of its comprehensive coverage I feel it will be of use to the many other professional groups involved in the area of occupational health and safety such as occupational nurses, hygienists and safety officers all of whom have their own vocational qualifications and examinations. Medical students who encounter occupational medicine as part of their medical school curriculum may also find it of interest.

It is hoped that readers will not only be tested on their knowledge of the subject but that they will also be stimulated to pursue further reading on the topics covered, both of which should contribute to examination success.

I wish to thank my colleagues, former tutors, and examiners who have contributed directly or indirectly to the preparation of this book. In particular, I would to thank Patricia Duffy and Linda Boyd for their help and dedication in the preparation of the text.

KA
Belfast

Introduction

Multiple choice questions (MCQs) have become an established and recognized method of assessing a wide range of facts and concepts in many postgraduate examinations. Candidates find answering MCQs to be a useful means of revision because they provide a broad test of basic knowledge across a syllabus. For this reason students preparing for non-MCQ examinations will also find it worthwhile to test the depth and extent of their learning by the use of MCQs.

The technique of answering MCQs is important with individuals tending to develop their own approach which has, hopefully, evolved from previous success. However it is essential to read each question carefully, not to look unduly for abstruse meanings and if possible try and avoid overt guessing (this is particularly relevant in papers that are negatively marked, i.e. marks are deducted for incorrect answers).

For the purposes of using this book as a revision aid readers are recommended to refrain from using the 'don't know' response as far as possible and to try and commit themselves to making definite decisions on the anwsers.

The questions are of two basic types:

- One is the traditional MCQ where one or more of the listed responses may be true.
- The other is of the 'match the following' type – in this the reader is asked to match one of the responses to a particular question number. Only one response is correct for each question number.

Correct answers with explanations are given over the page from each set of questions. For more detailed accounts of the topics covered, I recommend that reference is made to one of the standard textbooks and indeed would suggest that the stimulation of such cross-reading is one of the benefits of this book.

History and development of occupational medicine

Match the following:

1. Georgius Agricola.
2. Bernadino Ramazzini.
3. Charles Turner Thackrah.
4. Thomas Percival.

a. *Health and Morals of Apprentices Act 1802.*
b. *Effects of the Principal Arts, Trades and Professions ... on Health and Longevity.*
c. *De Re Metallica.*
d. *De Morbis Artificum Diatriba.*

5. **Sir Thomas Legge:**
   a. Was the first medical inspector of factories.
   b. Is associated with five axioms for disease prevention.
   c. Produced acclaimed work in mercury poisoning.
   d. Was a seventeenth century physician.
   e. Introduced a convention on the content of paints for indoor use.

6. **In early health & safety legislation:**
   a. The *Factory Act of 1833* introduced medical certification of employed children.
   b. Notification was introduced in 1840.
   c. The *Factory Act of 1855* allowed certifying surgeons to investigate industrial accidents.
   d. Factory inspection systems were regionalized by the *Factories and Workshops Act (1878)*.
   e. The *Mines Act of 1842* addressed employment of women in mines.

Match the following: Established in:

7. Medical Inspectorate.   a. 1833

8. Examining Surgeon.   b. 1972

9. Factory Inspectorate.   c. 1937

10. Employment Medical Advisory Service.   d. 1898

1. c. 1494–1555. Wrote on foul air in metal mines in Bohemia. Recommended better ventilation and wearing of veils over the face. In 1556 published *De Re Metallica* – treatise on disease and accidents prevalent in miners.
2. d. 1663–1714. Professor of medicine in Padua and Madena. Known as the 'Father of occupational medicine'.
3. b. 1795–1833. Based in Leeds. This treatise is regarded as the first British textbook of occupational medicine.
4. a. 1774–1804. Produced a report which lead to *Health and Morals of Apprentices Act 1802* – regarded as the first factory act.
5. a. True
   b. True
   c. False Did acclaimed work on lead poisoning.
   d. False Appointed as the first of Her Majesty's Medical Inspectors of Factories in 1898.
   e. False Resigned in 1919 due to the Government's failure to introduce an international convention banning white lead in paint for indoor use.
6. a. True
   b. False The *Factory Act of 1898*.
   c. True   Certifying surgeons investigated industrial accidents and certified young people as being fit for work.
   d. False This centralized the system of inspection with a Chief Inspector based in London.
   e. True   It prohibited the employment of women (and boys under the age of 10) at the pit face.
7. d.
8. c. *Factory Act 1937*. Carried out pre-employment and periodic examinations of young persons and adults in certain trades under the supervision of Medical Inspectors of Factories.
9. a. Set up by the *Factory Act 1833*.
10. b. EMAS is a division of the Health and Safety Executive. It advises employers, trade unions, doctors working in industry, individual employees and the self-employed on occupational health matters.

Legal issues

11. *Health and Safety at Work Act (HSAWA) 1974*:
    a. Covers all people at work.
    b. Puts a duty on employees to ensure safe/healthy working conditions.
    c. Is enforced by the HSC (Health and Safety Commission).
    d. Requires a written safety policy to be drawn up.
    e. Is an example of common law.

12. **Enforcement of *HSAWA 1974* can include:**
    a. Improvement notices.
    b. Codes of practice.
    c. Prohibition notices.
    d. Injunction notices.
    e. Barring orders.

13. *Control of Substances Hazardous to Health (COSHH) Regulations*:
    a. Replaced the *HSAWA 1974*.
    b. Exclude substances with an MEL or OES.
    c. Emphasize a need for training and education of employees.
    d. Include lead and asbestos.
    e. Exclude ionizing radiations.

NOTE: MEL = Maximum Exposure Limit
OES = Occupational Exposure Standard

Legal issues

11.
- a. True — *HSAWA* provides the legal basis for controlling working conditions in the UK and is an example of enabling legislation.
- b. False — It is the employers duty to provide safe and healthy working conditions.
- c. False — Enforcement is the responsibility of the Health and Safety Executive (HSE). Local authorities carry out responsibilities in relation to environmental matters.
- d. True
- e. False — It is an example of statute law, i.e. passed by an Act of Parliament.

12.
- a. True — Usually issued if there is a breach of the *HSAWA* and the employer is given a period of time to comply.
- b. True — These can be 'approved' where failure to observe is a criminal offence or 'unapproved' where failure to observe is not deemed to be a criminal offence.
- c. True — Prohibition notices can be 'immediate' or 'deferred'.
- d. False
- e. False

13.
- a. False — *COSHH Regulations* are enacted under the *HSAWA 1974*.
- b. False — Includes virtually all chemical and microbiological substances likely to be encountered in the workplace (including those with OES and MEL).
- c. True
- d. False — Lead and asbestos are covered by approved codes of practice.
- e. True — Ionizing radiation is also covered by an approved code of practice.

Legal issues

14. **Which of the following is not associated with *COSHH*:**
    a. Assessment.
    b. Control.
    c. Health surveillance.
    d. Access to personal computerized records.
    e. Statutory rules for packaging and labelling of containers.

15. **The 'six pack' EU directives:**
    a. Covered health and safety management.
    b. Set out broad duties to assess risk.
    c. Included vibration and EM radiation.
    d. Replaced *COSHH Regulations*.
    e. Are the result of ILO recommendations.

16. **The *Management of Health and Safety at Work Regulations 1992* (Management Regulations):**
    a. Set out duties that apply to a limited number of workplaces.
    b. Encourage a systematic approach to health and safety management.
    c. Deal with competent persons and emergency procedures.
    d. Do not cover temporary workers.
    e. Only apply to companies employing five or more persons.

NOTE: EU = European Union
EM = Electromagnetic
ILO = International Labour Organization

17. **The *Manual Handling Operations Regulations 1992*:**
    a. Only apply to weights in excess of 10 kg.
    b. Exclude pushing operations using wheeled trolleys.
    c. Replace old regulations with a modern ergonomic approach.
    d. Involve an assessment of all manual handling operations.
    e. Specify dimensions of containers to be lifted by hand.

Legal issues

14. a. False   *COSHH Regulations* are essentially designed to ensure that an employer carries out a risk assessment if engaged in work that may expose employees to substances hazardous to health. There is a duty to control exposure and monitor the environment.
    b. False
    c. False   Health surveillance may be indicated. Provision for education and training of employees must be made.
    d. True   Although records must be kept for defined periods.
    e. True

15. a. True   The *Management of Health and Safety at Work Regulations*.
    b. True
    c. False   These are included in a proposed *Physical Agents Directive*.
    d. False
    e. False   They are derived from the EU *Framework Directive on Health and Safety at Work (1989)*.

16. a. False   It sets out broad duties that apply to almost all workplaces.
    b. True
    c. True   'Competent persons' are required to help devise and apply measures to allow compliance under health and safety legislation.
    d. False   Temporary workers must be provided with health and safety information to meet their needs.
    e. False   No limits applied.

17. a. False   No specific requirements on weight limits are set.
    b. False   Includes lifting, pushing, carrying or moving a load whether by hand or use of other bodily force.
    c. True
    d. True   The ergonomic assessment involves the load, the task, the working environment and an individual's capabilities.
    e. False   Not specified.

Legal issues

18. In the *Workplace (Health, Safety and Welfare) Regulations 1992*:
    a. Construction sites and mines are included.
    b. Four broad areas of working environment, safety, facilities and housekeeping are covered.
    c. Agricultural premises distant from main buildings are exempt.
    d. Only the occupier of a building has duties under the terms of the Regulations.
    e. First-aid provision in the workplace is a consideration.

19. The *Provision and Use of Work Equipment Regulations 1992*: PUWER
    a. Include machines of all kinds excluding hand tools.
    b. Exclude installing and dismantling of equipment.
    c. Place a duty on employers to ensure equipment is maintained and in efficient working order.
    d. List requirements for work equipment to deal with selected hazards.
    e. Advise that equipment complies with EU product safety directives.

20. *Personal Protective Equipment (PPE) at Work Regulations 1992*:
    a. Take precedence over *COSHH* and *Noise at Work Regulations*.
    b. Include PPE used for road transport.
    c. Specify that training, information and instruction should be given to employees.
    d. Define suitable PPE.
    e. State all PPE must have a 'CE' mark.

NOTE: CE = European Union Safety Standard Mark

Legal issues

18.
- a. False — Excluded are means of transport, construction sites and mines.
- b. True — 'Facilities' include toilets, washrooms, clothing stores and rest areas.
- c. False — These are exempt from most of the Regulations but those relating to toilets, drinking water and washing facilities apply.
- d. False — For example, the owner of a building also has duties under the Regulations.
- e. False — Existing first-aid regulations apply (*Health and Safety (First-Aid) Regulations 1981*).

19.
- a. False — Applies a broad definition to 'work equipment' which is deemed to be everything from a hand tool to a complete plant.
- b. False — 'Use of work equipment' includes installing and dismantling as well as starting, stopping, repairing, transporting, etc.
- c. True — And suitable for intended use.
- d. True — For example, to provide machine guards, protect against breakage, rupture, fire, explosion, etc.
- e. True

20.
- a. False — Does not apply where *COSHH* or *Noise at Work Regulations* apply.
- b. False — Excluded are safety helmets for road transport use, sports equipment, and ordinary working clothes and uniforms.
- c. True — Also need to carry out assessments of risks and of PPE intended for use.
- d. True — This is appropriate for the risks and working conditions, takes account of workers' needs and fits properly.
- e. False — Possession of CE mark is not a necessity for PPE under this directive.

Legal issues

21. **In the *Health and Safety (Display Screen Equipment) Regulations 1992*:**
    a. Display screen equipment (DSE) workstations have to be assessed.
    b. Users of DSE are entitled to eyesight tests.
    c. Laptop computers are exempt.
    d. Work activity should be planned.
    e. Tinted glasses can be provided if desired.

22. **The EU *Biological Agents Directive*:**
    a. Will be introduced as a schedule of *COSHH*.
    b. Classifies biological agents into four hazard categories.
    c. Does not encompass vaccination of workers.
    d. Advises that lists of exposed employees must be kept.
    e. Applies to immediate exposure but not delayed.

23. **The following statements with regard to the EU *Pregnant Workers Directive* are correct:**
    a. Applies only during pregnancy.
    b. Female employees must notify employers of their condition in writing.
    c. Night work is prohibited for pregnant workers.
    d. Entitlement to suspension from work at normal rate of pay.
    e. Health and safety provisions of the Directive are implemented by an amendment of the 'Management Regulations'.

Legal issues

21. a. True — This is to ensure workstations satisfy minimum requirements as far as the DSE, desk, chair, working environment, task design and software are concerned.
b. True — Users are entitled to appropriate eye and eyesight tests and to special glasses if needed solely for DSE work.
c. False — Portable systems are exempt only if not in prolonged use.
d. True — Planning should ensure breaks or changes in activity.
e. False

22. a. True — A 'biological agent' is any micro-organism, cell culture or human endoparasite which may cause infection, allergy, toxicity or other hazard to human health.
b. True — According to severity of effect on health.
c. False — If a risk is present and a vaccine exists there is a duty to inform employees and offer the vaccination.
d. True
e. False — Both types of exposure are covered by the regulations.

23. a. False — Also applies to women who have recently given birth and are breast feeding.
b. True
c. False — Only prohibited if it is a threat to health.
d. True — If it is not possible to avoid a risk to health by offering suitable alternative work.
e. True — These include risk assessments, avoidance measures and preventive actions including alternatives to working conditions or hours of work.

Legal issues

24. **With regard to the *Chemicals (Hazard Information and Packaging for Supply) Regulations (CHIP) 1994*:**
    a. The transport of dangerous substances is covered.
    b. Information to be included in safety data sheets is specified.
    c. Suppliers are responsible for the safe and suitable packaging of substances.
    d. Include ionizing radiation in their schedules.
    e. Tactile warnings are required for the benefit of blind persons.

24. a. False *CHIP 1994* deals only with the supply of dangerous substances or preparations.
   b. True Set out a series of headings.
   c. True
   d. False Do not include any substance which is dangerous for supply covered by *Ionizing Radiation Regulations 1985*.
   e. True For substances labelled 'very toxic', 'toxic', 'corrosive', 'harmful', 'extremely flammable' or 'highly flammable'.

Occupational hygiene

Match the following:

25. Occupational hygiene.
26. Hazard.
27. Risk.
28. OES (occupational exposure standard).
29. OEL (occupational exposure limit)

a. Substance with potential to cause harm.
b. Relates to adequate control of substances for *COSHH*.
c. Level to which employees can be exposed without harming their health.
d. Likelihood of harm occurring in conditions of use of a substance.
e. Science and practice of protecting health of persons at work by controlling their exposure to workplace hazards.

What are the following used to measure:

30. Draeger tube.
31. Kata thermometer.
32. Whirling hygrometer.
33. Pump operated personal sampler.
34. Globe thermometer.

a. Air humidity.
b. Sampling of gases, vapours and dusts.
c. Radiant temperature.
d. Location sampling of gases and vapours.
e. Air velocity.

Match the following to the units of measurement:

35. Noise.
36. Airborne concentration of dusts.
37. Vapour concentration in air.
38. Asbestos dust.
39. Ionizing radiation.

a. mg/m^3.
b. ppm.
c. dB.
d. sievert.
e. fibres/ml.

Occupational hygiene

25. e. The essential steps involve, anticipation, recognition; evaluation, and control of the hazard.

26. a.

27. d.

28. c. Previously known as TLVs. Represent a level to which an employee can be exposed without harming their health. There are two types of OES: an OEL (occupational exposure limit) and an MEL (maximal exposure limit).

29. b. OEL can be long term, i.e. over an eight-hour period, expressed as a time weighted average (TWA) or short term, usually ten minutes (STEL).

30. d. This is a detector tube that contains a chemical reagent which produces a colour change when a contaminated air sample is drawn through it.

31. e. This is a liquid filled thermometer with a large silvered bulb and a smaller bulb. It measures the cooling power of air and using a formula the air velocity can be calculated.

32. a. Contains a wet and dry bulb – the difference in readings is used to calculate the humidity of the air.

33. b. Usually used to monitor levels of dust or vapour in the worker's breathing zone.

34. c.

35. c. Decibel is a measure of sound intensity expressed on a logarithmic scale.

36. a.

37. b.

38. e.

39. d. The sievert is an expression of the dose equivalent and is an index of the risk of harm following exposure to ionizing radiation.

Occupational hygiene

40. The following statements with regard to the aerodynamic diameter of particles are correct:
   a. It is that of a theoretical sphere of unit density with the same air speed characteristics as a particle under investigation.
   b. Inhalable into the nose between 100 μm–1000 μm in diameter.
   c. Inhalable to bronchus and bronchioles between 25 μm–50 μm in diameter.
   d. Inhalable (respirable) to alveoli if less than 7 μm in diameter.
   e. In fibres the length is more important than diameter in determining respirability.

41. Control of exposure by ventilation:
   a. Is preferable to total enclosure.
   b. Separates the worker from hazard by surrounding his breathing zone with good quality air.
   c. Is better if designed and installed in the initial building stage of a plant.
   d. Uses dilution ventilation for substances with moderate to high toxicity.
   e. Employs local exhaust ventilation to capture contaminants at source.

42. With regard to personal protective equipment:
   a. 'Nominal Protection Factor' is the ratio of contamination outside a face mask to that inside.
   b. Problems with face masks include poor user technique.
   c. Usefulness of gloves is related to breakthrough time and permeation rates.
   d. PVC gloves allow greater sensitivity than rubber gloves.
   e. Effectiveness of hearing protectors is defined in terms of attenuated protection levels.

43. The following statements with regard to walk-through surveys are correct:
   a. Carried out by observing the working environment.
   b. Detailed checklists are required.
   c. Anticipation of potential problems is a key activity.
   d. Allow possible hazards to be identified.
   e. Can only be undertaken by skilled hygienists.

40. a. True
 b. False — Particles between 50 μm–100 μm are inhalable into the nose.
 c. False — 8 μm–20 μm.
 d. True
 e. False — A respirable fibre is greater than 5 μm in length with a length:breadth ratio of 3:1 and a diameter less than 3 μm. The diameter is the determining factor.

41. a. False — Total enclosure of a hazardous process is preferable to general ventilation.
 b. True — And removes vitiated air.
 c. True — More cost effective and usually more efficient if properly planned.
 d. False — As it dilutes the concentration of contaminants in the air it is only suitable for substances of low toxicity.
 e. True — And conveys them away via a ducting system.

42. a. True
 b. True — Breaks around the face seal, filter blockage, poor fit and facial hair also contribute to the problems.
 c. True — Technical advice from the manufacturer will also help.
 d. False — It is to an extent the fit rather than the material which is important in terms of 'feel'.
 e. False — Effectiveness of hearing protectors is defined in terms of 'assumed protection level' at the wearers ear to below Lep'd of 90 dB(A).

43. a. True
 b. False — Do not need to be detailed. However they need to cover main headings of areas to be assessed.
 c. True — Anticipating potential problems as a consequence of the working environment is very important.
 d. True — And hence eliminated or modified.
 e. False — Walk-through surveys can be usefully carried out by practitioners with basic OH knowledge using their skills in a critical and evaluating manner.

Occupational hygiene

44. Risk assessment:
   a. Is an examination of the workplace to see what could cause harm and what precautions are needed to prevent harm occurring.
   b. Needs to be carried out by a certified risk-assessor.
   c. Requires written records to be kept for companies with greater than ten employees.
   d. Obliges the employer to be able to show how it was carried out.
   e. Has the key steps of recognition, evaluation, control and review.

44. a. True
b. False — Can be carried out by a responsible, competent person, e.g. a safety officer or safety representative.
c. False — Written records are required if companies have five or more employees.
d. False — Do not need to be provided if it can be shown a proper examination took place and the outcome was reasonable in terms of precautions and level of risk.
e. True — It is important to review a risk assessment periodically, particularly if new equipment or significant changes to working practices are introduced.

Physical hazards

Noise

45. In the properties of sound:
   a. The human ear can hear in the range of 20 Hz–20 kHz.
   b. An octave band is a frequency interval where the top f is four times that of the bottom f.
   c. The decibel scale is a logarithmic scale of sound frequency.
   d. A 10 dB increase represents a sound twice as loud.
   e. A 3 dB increase in noise level results in halving the allowable exposure time.

46. In noise-induced hearing loss:
   a. A familial type of hearing loss may cause a 4 kHz dip.
   b. The characteristics of the noise are important.
   c. Individual variation or susceptibility does not apply.
   d. Ototoxic drugs and age changes do not cause a noise-induced hearing loss pattern.
   e. Duration of exposure is important.

Match the following:

47. dB(A)   a. Depends on level of noise and exposure time.

48. Lep'd.   b. 140 dB.

49. 2nd action level.   c. Noise weighting that closely simulates the human ear.

50. Noise dose.   d. Level of daily continual personal exposure.

51. Peak action level.   e. Hearing protection mandatory.

Physical hazards

45. a. True   This range is for young persons.
     b. False   An octave band is a frequency interval where the top f is double the bottom f.
     c. False   A logarithmic scale of sound intensity.
     d. True   A 10 dB increase represents a sound twice as loud but a ten fold increase in sound energy.
     e. True   Known as the '3 dB rule'.

46. a. True   An autosomal dominant hearing loss in the range 3 kHz–6 kHz.
     b. True   Impact noise may affect 6 kHz more than other frequencies. The maximum effect of single frequency noise is usually one half of an octave band above that frequency.
     c. False
     d. False   They may do and may show a 4 kHz loss.
     e. True

47. c. Good correlation between dB(A) levels and risk of noise-induced deafness and annoyance of noise.

48. d. Is used to represent personal exposure over an eight-hour period. Also known as Leq(8h) and Lex(8h).

49. e. Lep'd of 90dB(A). The level below which noise should be reduced if possible.

50. a. Can be used to calculate Lep'd.

51. b. A sudden very loud or impact noise.

Physical hazards

52. In occupational deafness:
   a. There is a classical 2 kHz dip.
   b. A large degree of recovery is possible if removed from exposure.
   c. Pure tone audiometry is used for assessment.
   d. A loss of at least 50 dB in each ear is a prescribed disease.
   e. Tinnitus is an early warning sign.

53. A hearing conservation programme involves:
   a. A noise survey and designation of hearing protection zones.
   b. Engineering control measures to reduce noise levels at source.
   c. Total enclosure of all sound sources greater than 90 dB(A).
   d. Twice yearly employee audiometry.
   e. Continuing education.

54. The following are associated with sensorineural deafness:
   a. Rubella syndrome.
   b. Acoustic neuroma.
   c. Otosclerosis.
   d. Paget's disease.
   e. Presbyacusis.

Vibration

55. Vibration:
   a. Is measured in terms of frequency and acceleration.
   b. Is covered by the EU *Physical Agents Directive*.
   c. Of the whole body type may lead to ischaemia of feet.
   d. Has a critical range for segmental vibration of 8–1400 Hz.
   e. May cause multi-system effects in the body.

Physical hazards

52.
- a. False — There is a classical 4 kHz dip.
- b. False — If damage is severe recovery does not take place and may progress despite removal from exposure.
- c. True — The subject should not have been exposed to loud noise for up to twelve hours prior to the test.
- d. True — Substantial sensorineural hearing loss amounting to at least 50 dB in each ear, being due in the case of at least one ear, to occupational noise and being the average of pure tone losses measured by audiometry over 1, 2 and 3 kHz frequencies.
- e. False — Difficulty hearing conversation against a noisy background is usually the presenting complaint. Tinnitus, if present at all, would be a late symptom.

53.
- a. True
- b. True
- c. False — 90 dB(A) is the second action level (*Noise at Work Regulations 1989*) and hearing protection is mandatory at this level.
- d. False — Audiometry should be baseline or pre-employment and after that dependent on level of noise exposure but probably annually for two years and then every two to three years after that.
- e. True — To promote understanding of and compliance with hearing conservation measures.

54.
- a. True
- b. True
- c. False — Conductive deafness.
- d. False — Associated with conductive deafness.
- e. True

55.
- a. True
- b. True
- c. False — May get symptoms of back pain, general fatigue and stress.
- d. True — Segmental vibration represents vibration to specific parts of the body such as the hand or arm.
- e. True — These may be vascular, neurological and musculoskeletal.

Physical hazards

56. Hand–arm vibration syndrome (HAVS):
   a. Is a chronic progressive disorder with a latent period of one to fifteen years.
   b. Is a prescribed industrial disease.
   c. Causes damage to digital nerves and arteries.
   d. Is classified using the Copenhagen scale.
   e. Does not involve the thumbs.

57. The differential diagnosis of HAVS commonly includes:
   a. Primary Raynaud's disease.
   b. Costo-clavicular syndrome.
   c. Systemic lupus erythematosus.
   d. Carpal tunnel syndrome.
   e. Osteoarthritis

58. In the management of HAVS the following are correct:
   a. Each hand is assessed separately.
   b. Doppler Finger Blood Flow readings are diagnostic.
   c. Stellate ganglion blocks are a first line treatment.
   d. Engineering controls are used to reduce or avoid exposure to vibration.
   e. Cold exposure and smoking should be avoided.

Light

59. Visibility of a task depends on:
   a. Luminance of the task.
   b. Visual fringing.
   c. Luminance of the background.
   d. Contrast.
   e. Colour flickering.

Physical hazards

56. a. True   Prevalence and severity increase as the vibration intensity and exposure duration increase.
     b. False   Vibration white finger is a prescribed industrial disease.
     c. True   There is occlusion of proximal segments of digital arteries which reduces the size of the lumen.
     d. False   It is the 'Stockholm Scale'.
     e. False   Vibration white finger can involve the thumbs.

57. a. True   Here the finger blanching is usually bilateral extending to the finger base with other abnormally cold extremities, e.g. feet and ears.
     b. True
     c. True
     d. True
     e. False   Rheumatoid arthritis.

58. a. True
     b. False   This test may be used but is not diagnostic.
     c. False   Can be used as a special treatment to improve circulation however results overall are not good.
     d. True
     e. True

59. a. True
     b. False
     c. True
     d. True
     e. False   Flickering may cause symptoms of visual fatigue.

Match the following:

60. Illuminance. a. Power of a source to emit light.
61. Luminous intensity. b. Luminous flux reflected: luminous flux incident.
62. Luminance. c. The intensity of light falling on a surface.
63. Reflectance. d. The light emitted by a source or received by a surface.
64. Luminous flux. e. The physical brightness of a surface.

Radiation

Match the following:

65. Beta particles. a. Cannot penetrate the skin.
66. Radioactivity. b. Very penetrative and very hazardous.
67. Ionization. c. Spontaneous process of decay.
68. Gamma rays. d. Radiations which release electrically charged particles in tissues.
69. Alpha particles. e. Can penetrate skin to 1 cm and are hazardous to superficial tissues.

70. The following statements with regard to ionizing radiation are correct:
    a. Tissues with rapidly dividing cells are most sensitive.
    b. An example of a stochastic effect is a cataract.
    c. Deterministic effects vary according to dose.
    d. Statutory dose limits are to prevent stochastic effects.
    e. A sievert is a unit of dose equivalence.

Physical hazards

60. c. Unit of measurement is 'lux' which is lumen per m^2.

61. a. Unit of measurement is 'candela'.

62. e. Unit of measurement is 'candela per m^2'.

63. b.

64. d. Unit of measurement is 'lumen'.

65. e. Two types, electrons with a negative charge and positrons with a positive charge. They pose a problem to skin and subcutaneous tissues and to internal organs if ingested or inhaled into the body.

66. c. Decay means the unstable nature of certain atomic nuclei emitting charged particles, electromagnetic waves or neutrons to allow adoption of a more stable state.

67. d.

68. b. Are a form of electromagnetic radiation.

69. a. Are positively charged. Have difficulty penetrating the dead outer layer of skin. Do not represent a significant hazard unless absorbed into the body (e.g. by ingestion, inhalation or wound contamination).

70. a. True   Such as lymphocytes, gonads, bone marrow, intestinal lining and epidermis.
    b. False Stochastic effects are those such as carcinogenesis and genetic damage. They are dose related but there is no threshold level for these effects.
    c. True   Also known as non-stochastic. An example is acute radiation syndrome. The severity of effect is a function of the radiation dose exceeding a threshold level. Cataract is an example of a delayed non-stochastic or deterministic effect.
    d. False Limits are set to prevent non-stochastic effects as these have a threshold. The possibility of stochastic effects are limited by keeping all exposures to radiation as low as reasonably achievable.
    e. True   The absorbed dose in Grays multiplied by a factor to take account of the type of radiation (this factor is known as the 'relative biological effectiveness').

Physical hazards

71. **With regard to ionizing radiation the following are true:**
    a. Acute radiation syndrome develops following whole body irradiation of 2 Sv or more.
    b. Background radiation is around 10 mSv per year.
    c. Threshold for skin damage is 3 Sv acute or 0.5 Sv per year.
    d. ICRP dose limit for pregnant women is 10 mSv per year.
    e. Classified workers are those liable to receive in excess of three tenths of annual dose limits.

NOTE: ICRP = International Commission on Radiological Protection

72. **Features of ultra-violet radiation are:**
    a. It is divided into two wavelengths.
    b. UV(A) produces serious effects on the skin and cornea.
    c. Eyes may develop a tolerance to exposure.
    d. Over exposure may lead to cataract formation.
    e. UV(B) is associated with snow-blindness.

73. **Features of infra-red radiation are:**
    a. Three wavelengths.
    b. Severe skin burns.
    c. Injuries to the lens and retina.
    d. IR(A) is normally visible.
    e. A recognized hazard of glass blowing.

74. **Features of microwave radiation are:**
    a. It is at the high end of the electromagnetic spectrum.
    b. It is linked to eye damage.
    c. Pulsed waves are more damaging than continuous emissions.
    d. Carcinogenicity in humans.
    e. Skin burns due to local irradiation.

75. **The following statements with regard to lasers are correct:**
    a. They emit light of different wavelengths depending on the type of laser.
    b. It is safe to view their reflections without the need for eye protection.
    c. Class 1 lasers cause skin burns.
    d. They may pose a fire risk.
    e. The main risk to the eye is cataract formation.

Physical hazards

71.
  a. True — In a single dose or over a short period.
  b. False — In the UK it is 1 mSv per year but may vary depending on location in the country.
  c. True
  d. True — Furthermore for women of reproductive capacity the abdominal dose limit is 13 mSv in any consecutive three month interval.
  e. True — Are required to undergo pre-employment and annual review examinations.

72.
  a. False — Three wavelengths UV(A): 315–400 nm, UV(B): 280–315 nm and UV(C): 100–280 nm. UV(C) is mostly absorbed in the atmosphere.
  b. False — UV(B) does this and is associated with photokeratitis of arc eye. Most of the UV(B) is filtered by the cornea.
  c. False — Eye protection must always be worn.
  d. True — Usually associated with UV(A) as most of this is absorbed in the lens.
  e. True

73.
  a. True — IR(A): 760–1400 nm, IR(B): 1400–3000 nm and IR(C): 3000 nm–1 mm
  b. False — Skin can burn but relative slow heating allows withdrawal from the exposure to take place.
  c. True — Causing cataract formation.
  d. False — It is normally invisible although some may perceive a dull red glow.
  e. True — Due to IR(A) radiation – glass blowers cataract.

74.
  a. False — It is at the low end with wavelength range 1 nm–1 m.
  b. True — Cataract formation.
  c. True
  d. False — No sound evidence to confirm this.
  e. True

75.
  a. True — There are four classes based on their type and energy emmission. Class 4 is the most powerful.
  b. False — Reflections of Classes 1–3 are safe to view however those of class 4 are not.
  c. False — Class 1 are low powered and do not cause skin burns.
  d. True — Only Class 4.
  e. False — Main risk is a retinal burn.

Temperature

Match the following:

76. Convection.
77. Thermoregulatory mechanisms.
78. Radiation.
79. Evaporation.
80. Effective temperature index.

a. Does not depend on air movement.
b. A measure of temperature, humidity and air velocity.
c. Dependent on air temperature and velocity.
d. Peripheral vasodilatation and sweating.
e. Dependent on temperature, humidity and air velocity.

81. In heat-induced disorders:
a. Heat stroke is associated with hyperpyrexia, hot dry skin and mental disturbance.
b. Heat stress may be a feature of mining, iron and steel industry and glass-making.
c. Salt and water balance is important exclusively in outdoor work.
d. Heat syncope is a relatively common component and is due to vasodilatation.
e. Treatment of heat stroke involves slow cooling.

82. With regard to a cold environment the following are true:
a. Wind chill index is the cooling power of cool air and air movement on exposed skin expressed in unit time.
b. In hypothermia the core temperature is 35°C or less.
c. Presence or absence of moisture is not important.
d. Worker selection for cold conditions excludes diabetes and hypothyroidism.
e. Frost bite, frost nip and chilblains are all examples of local hazards of cold exposure.

Physical hazards

76. c. Surface area is also important.

77. d.

78. a. Depends on the difference between temperature of skin or clothing and the surrounding surfaces (e.g. walls, machinery, etc.).

79. e.

80. b. This index gives a measure of the warmth of the environment.

81. a. True Associated with body temperature of 41°C and above. May lead to unconsciousness/convulsions and death.
    b. True Also known as heat cramps.
    c. False
    d. True Poor physical fitness and lack of acclimatization to the work are contributory factors.
    e. False Treatment of heat stroke involves rapid cooling.

82. a. True
    b. True
    c. False Presence of moisture in cold conditions increases the amount of heat loss.
    d. False Considerations include mobility, Raynaud's disease, history of chilblains or other cold injuries amongst others.
    e. True

Compressed air and diving

83. The following statements with regard to decompression sickness are correct:
   a. Only occurs in workers exposed to helium at high pressures.
   b. 'Niggles' and 'bends' are examples of Type 1 symptoms.
   c. 'Chokes' and 'staggers' are related to Type 2 symptoms.
   d. Aseptic bone necrosis occurs at the proximal end of phalanges.
   e. Incidence is about 10–12 per cent of all decompressions.

84. In medical assessments for diving:
   a. A certificate of fitness is required bi-annually.
   b. Peptic ulcer, hernia and obesity are deterrents to employment.
   c. Personal medical records are held by divers.
   d. A dental assessment is important.
   e. Assessments are laid down by *COSHH Regulations*.

Physical hazards

83. a. False   Can occur in anyone exposed to air or other gases at increased pressures (e.g. divers, compressed air workers).
    b. True   Type 1 symptoms are mainly peripheral effects. 'Niggles' consists of pruritus with limb discomfort. The 'bends' is associated with extreme limb pain. Both may exhibit skin mottling.
    c. True   Type 2 symptoms are more generalized and severe. 'Chokes' relates to dyspnoea and 'staggers' to vertigo.
    d. False   Thought to be due to infarction secondary to nitrogen emboli in arterial vessels of bone. The distal end of femur, proximal ends of tibia and humerus are common sites.
    e. False   Incidence is thought to vary from less than 1 per cent to 2 per cent of total decompressions. The majority of cases of decompression sickness are of Type 1, i.e. the less serious.

84. a. False   Annually.
    b. True
    c. True
    d. True   Due to potential air entrapment in dental caries.
    e. False   *Medical Code of Practice for Work in Compressed Air* and *Diving Operations at Work Regulations 1981*.

Respiratory disorders

85. With regard to respiratory function tests the following are true:
 a. Can be used to monitor exposure to dusts and other materials known to affect the lungs.
 b. FEV% can be used to distinguish between obstructive and restrictive airways disease.
 c. Peak expiratory flow rate is useful in monitoring late effects of restrictive airflow disease.
 d. Gas transfer factor is a useful test in reversible airways obstruction.
 e. Serial peak flow measurements are useful in monitoring exposure to asbestos.

86. In coal worker's pneumoconiosis the following are correct:
 a. Coal dust can be a mixture of coal, kaolin, mica and silica.
 b. Rounded opacities, progressive massive fibrosis and cavitation are found in the lungs.
 c. Rounded opacities, graded by ILO classification, are predominant in lower lobes.
 d. Haemoptysis is a characteristic sign.
 e. Has an association with rheumatoid arthritis.

87. In silicosis:
 a. The diatomite form is most common.
 b. Eggshell calcification occurs in periphery of hilar nodes.
 c. Finger clubbing is an early manifestation.
 d. Opacities predominate in upper lobes.
 e. There is a predisposition to tuberculosis.

88. With regard to asbestosis:
 a. Chrysotile is the commonest form of asbestos used commercially.
 b. Is an association with tuberculosis.
 c. Fibrosis of upper lobes is usual.
 d. Finger clubbing is a late sign.
 e. As an association mesothelioma is commonly found in the peritoneum.

85. a. True
    b. True
    c. False   Useful in monitoring reversible airways obstruction.
    d. False   Tests of gas transfer or exchange are not suitable for routine purposes. They are usually used to assess restrictive type lung diseases.
    e. False   Obstruction in asbestosis is unusual and hence serial peak flow monitoring would not be beneficial.

86. a. True
    b. True
    c. False   Rounded opacities have a preponderance for the upper lobes.
    d. False   Not usually present unless associated with coincidental chronic bronchitis, superimposed tuberculosis or progressive massive fibrosis.
    e. True   Caplan's syndrome.

87. a. False   This type of silicosis is rare.
    b. True   Seen on radiography.
    c. False   Finger clubbing not associated with uncomplicated cases.
    d. True   Pathology reveals connective tissue nodules in a 'whorled' pattern.
    e. True

88. a. True   Also known as 'white asbestos'.
    b. False   No association with TB. There is one with bronchogenic carcinoma – more likely in smokers.
    c. False   Changes more common in lower lobes.
    d. True
    e. False   Is usually associated with crocidolite exposure and principally affects the pleura.

89. **Byssinosis has the following features:**
    a. Caused by exposure to dust of cotton, flax, soft hemp and sisal.
    b. Characteristic mid-week chest tightness.
    c. Wheeze is common.
    d. The dust most hazardous in the aetiology is known as 'fly'.
    e. Can lead to irreversible airways obstruction.

90. **The following statements with regard to berylliosis are correct:**
    a. Get sarcoid-like granulomatous lesions in lungs.
    b. Finger clubbing is not a feature.
    c. Large opacities mainly in the lower lobes.
    d. A positive Kveim test.
    e. X-ray changes can resolve spontaneously.

91. **With regard to extrinsic allergic alveolitis the following are true:**
    a. Involves a Type 4 cell mediated hypersensitivity reaction.
    b. Most common form is farmers' lung.
    c. Symptoms may be progressive leading to irreversible airways obstruction.
    d. Get characteristic lower lobe shadowing.
    e. The antigen is typically a fungal protein.

92. **Fibrosing alveolitis is characterized by:**
    a. Finger clubbing.
    b. Decreased FEV/FVC ratio.
    c. Arterial $PaCO_2$ is reduced.
    d. Haemoptysis.
    e. Decreased residual volume.

93. **Features of asthma are:**
    a. Non-reactive airways.
    b. Reversible airways obstruction.
    c. Inflammatory changes in airways.
    d. FEV1 is significantly reduced in acute attacks.
    e. RAST may be used in evaluation.

Respiratory disorders

89. a. True
b. False — Usually first day back at work after a break such as a weekend or holiday. Thus typically a 'Monday morning tightness'.
c. False — May progress to chronic cough and progressive dyspnoea. Wheeze is not normally a feature.
d. False — 'Fly' is made of long cotton fibres up to 3 cm in length which are not inhalable. The fine cotton dust is the most hazardous.
e. True

90. a. True
b. False
c. False — Nodules of varying size can give a 'snowstorm appearance' with coalescence to form larger opacities – especially in the upper lobes.
d. False — The Kveim test is negative thus helping to differentiate it from sarcoidosis.
e. False

91. a. False — Is a Type 3 hypersensitivity reaction.
b. True — Bird fanciers' lung is also relatively common within this group of lung diseases.
c. False — Is an example of airways restriction primarily.
d. False — Shadowing and honeycombing are mostly in the upper lobes of chronic cases. In acute cases there may be a diffuse haze or widespread nodular shadowing.
e. True — In farmers' lung the causative agents are the spores of Microspora faeni and Thermoactinomyces vulgaris found in mouldy hay.

92. a. True — In advanced cases.
b. False — Ratio is normal.
c. True
d. False
e. True

93. a. False — They are hyper-reactive.
b. True — Although in some cases reversibility is not complete.
c. True — Particularly in its chronic form.
d. True — Degree of reduction dependent on severity.
e. True — Radioallergosorbent test (RAST) is a sero-analysis looking for specific IgE antibodies to inhalants thought to be allergens.

Respiratory disorders

94. In occupational asthma:
   a. There has been a decline in incidence over the past decade.
   b. The typical history is for symptoms to improve when away from work.
   c. There is an association with atopy in most cases.
   d. A persistent chronic condition can develop.
   e. Smoking increases the chances of contracting it.

95. Important causes of occupational asthma are:
   a. Di-isocyanates and epoxy resins.
   b. Cement.
   c. Colophony.
   d. Animal fur and dander.
   e. Detergents.

96. Chronic bronchitis has the following features:
   a. Chronic productive cough.
   b. Associated with prolonged exposure to bronchial irritants.
   c. FEV1/FVC ratio typically improves after bronchodilator inhalation.
   d. Physically demanding work may be difficult.
   e. Exercise programmes can be beneficial.

97. With regard to cigarette smoking:
   a. There is an increased risk of extrinsic allergic alveolitis in smokers.
   b. Cotton workers have a greater likelihood of developing bysinnosis if they smoke.
   c. The asbestos worker who smokes is more likely to contract mesothelioma.
   d. It is an important source of cadmium in the lung in the general population.
   e. Humidifier fever is less common in smokers.

98. With regard to metal fume fever the following are correct:
   a. It is commonly associated with zinc oxide fume.
   b. It is an example of a chemical pneumonitis.
   c. Pyrexia, malaise, dry cough and dyspnoea are typical.
   d. May progress to chronic bronchitis and emphysema.
   e. Repeated exposure may lead to limited tolerance.

Respiratory disorders

94. a. False   Approximately 500 new cases each year in the UK.
    b. True   In the early stages. This may not be so in established cases.
    c. False   Atopy may make some individuals more sensitive to a particular antigen but the role of atopy in causation of occupational asthma is not clearly established.
    d. True   In some cases removal from the source of exposure will not lead to complete resolution of asthma.
    e. True   Cigarette smoking increases the likelihood of sensitization.

95. a. True   See Appendix A.
    b. False   See Appendix A.
    c. True   See Appendix A.
    d. True   See Appendix A.
    e. True   Bacillus subtilis found in detergent manufacture.

96. a. True
    b. True
    c. False
    d. True
    e. True   Provided there is not severe heart disease.

97. a. False   The opposite seems to be true with non-smokers more likely to be affected.
    b. True
    c. False   Smoking increases the likelihood of developing lung cancer.
    d. True
    e. True   By a similar mechanism to that of extrinsic allergic alveolitis.

98. a. True   Also copper and magnesium. Less frequently with aluminium, cadmium, nickel, manganese and iron.
    b. False   Mechanism of the response is largely unknown.
    c. True
    d. False   Permanent pulmonary damage is rare.
    e. True   With characteristic recurrence on re-exposure after a period away from work (Monday fever).

Occupational dermatoses

Match the following:

99. Common cause of irritant contact dermatitis.
100. Oil folliculitis.
101. Occupational vitiligo.
102. Common cause of allergic contact dermatitis.
103. Chloracne.

a. Contact with polychlorinated aromatic hydrocarbons.
b. Hardwoods, epoxy resin, rubber, formaldehyde.
c. Result of irritation with mineral oil residues.
d. Detergents, solvents, cutting oils, cement.
e. Contact with alkyl phenols.

104. **Contact dermatitis:**
   a. May exhibit explosive onset.
   b. Shows an unusual distribution of eczema.
   c. Demonstrates a sustained response to topical steroid therapy.
   d. Does not improve away from work.
   e. Requires particular attention to the history.

Match the following:

105. A skin irritant.
106. Patch testing.
107. A skin allergen.
108. Photocontact dermatitis.
109. Contact urticaria.

a. Wheal and flare response sometimes found in hairdressers and animal handlers.
b. Provocation of contact dermatitis with stimulus of ultra-violet rays.
c. Use of test agents in allergic contact dermatitis.
d. An agent that directly damages cells if applied in sufficient concentration or for sufficient time.
e. An agent that induces a specific immunological sensitivity to itself.

Occupational dermatoses

99. d. See Appendix B.

100. c. Also known as oil acne. Can be caused by oils, pitch and tar. Greatest number are due to contact with mineral oils.

101. e. Use of a Woods lamp may help detect early cases.

102. b. See Appendix B.

103. a. Chloracne is a specific form of oil acne. The causative agents are known as 'chloracnegens'. There are cystic skin lesions with comedones, principally on the face and neck.

104. a. True
    b. True   Contact dermatitis principally affects hands (webs of fingers), forearms and face. The site is determined by what parts of the skin are exposed to the contact substance and may give a clue as to the cause.
    c. False Often have a failure of sustained response to topical steroid therapy.
    d. False The history, at least initially, is of an improvement when away from work.
    e. True   Taking a good history will often suggest a cause.

105. d. Irritants may be strong, e.g. acids, alkalis or solvents or weak, e.g. domestic detergents, oils and greases.

106. c. Standard batteries of antigens are used which include the suspect antigen.

107. e. Also known as a sensitizer. They elicit a Type 4 immunological reaction.

108. b. An example would be coal tar pitch and sunlight.

109. a. Occurs rapidly on application of substances to the skin, e.g. persulphates in hairdressing. May or may not have an immunological component to its aetiology. Heat, cold, mild trauma and sunlight may be a cause in some individuals.

Occupational dermatoses

110. **The following statements with regard to occupational dermatitis are correct:**
    a. Occupations associated with it include – engineering, hairdressing, woodworking and floristry.
    b. In general allergic contact dermatitis is commoner than irritant contact dermatitis.
    c. Previous history at pre-employment assessment is best indicator for future.
    d. For the employee personal economic issues can override preventive strategies.
    e. Widespread use of barrier creams have led to a decrease in the incidence.

111. **Workplace skin disease occurring in clusters may be due to:**
    a. Allergic contact dermatitis.
    b. Pityriasis rosea.
    c. A functional phenomenon.
    d. Photodermatitis.
    e. Vitiligo.

112. **In allergic contact dermatitis:**
    a. Skin which has been damaged is more likely to develop allergic contact dermatitis.
    b. Circulating IgE levels are high.
    c. The site of the rash tends to include secondary sites distant from that of the original contact.
    d. Atopy predisposes.
    e. May get cross-sensitization.

113. **In the management of dermatitis:**
    a. The acute case should be removed from the source of exposure.
    b. Alternative work will have to be found.
    c. A skin care policy may be of benefit.
    d. Cationic skin cleansers are the least likely to cause skin reactions.
    e. Solvents used as cleansers can be beneficial in removing oil and grease.

Occupational dermatoses

110.
a. True — See Appendix C.
b. False — Irritant contact dermatitis is in general more common.
c. True
d. True — This may be true if an individual is faced with moving to a less well paid job in order to avoid contact with an antigen. In other words the employee is likely to remain exposed rather than accept financial loss.
e. False — Use of these creams may raise general skin hygiene awareness within a workforce. Barrier creams may in themselves be a source of contact dermatitis in some sensitive individuals.

111.
a. True
b. False
c. True — Some individuals with pre-existing non-occupational skin disease may present as part of a 'cluster' of skin problems.
d. True
e. True — Occupational vitiligo may occur in clusters.

112.
a. True — For example damaged by abrasion, heat or degreasing solvents.
b. False — Is a Type 4 cell mediated reaction.
c. True — Particularly with progressive exposure to the allergen. The eyelids are frequently involved and in severe cases there is a generalized widespread rash.
d. False
e. True — Skin which is sensitized to a particular chemical may react to different but chemically similar substances.

113.
a. True — Treatment advised as necessary and advice given as to how further exposure can be avoided or reduced.
b. False — This is not necessary in all cases if, for example, certain agents can be substituted with less irritant or non-allergenic substances.
c. True — Stressing personal hygiene and providing good washing facilities and appropriate protective clothing.
d. False — Non-ionic are the least likely. Excessive use of skin cleansers should be avoided as they dry the skin.
e. False — Definitely not. Solvents used in this manner are a major cause of dermatitis.

114. With regard to psoriasis:
   a. It is characterized by dry, silvery scaling plaques and papules.
   b. Sero-positive arthritis is a feature.
   c. Occupational contact factors do not aggravate the condition.
   d. Pruritus is common.
   e. Catering work may be contraindicated.

Occupational dermatoses

114. a. True
 b. False Psoriatic arthropathy is not associated with presence of rheumatoid factor in the serum.
 c. False May be aggravated by physical or chemical trauma. The Koebner phenomenon is the appearance of lesions at the site of local trauma.
 d. False Rarely associated with itch.
 e. True If it involves exposed arms/forearms/scalp with shedding of scales which may be a source of staphylococcal infection.

Occupational cancers

115. **With regard to tumours of occupational origin the following are correct:**
    a. Probably account for around 3 per cent of all tumours.
    b. Usually have a short latent period.
    c. Deaths as a result may occur at a younger age.
    d. May occur in clusters.
    e. In the aetiology, repeated continuous exposure to a carcinogenic agent is crucial.

116. **In occupational cancer:**
    a. Carcinogenesis is a single-step process.
    b. Specific genes may be involved in the development of the condition.
    c. Organotrophy is the term used to describe carcinogenic genetic mutation.
    d. Metal salts account for most occupationally linked cancers.
    e. The Ames test is an in-vitro test of mutagenicity.

Match the following:

117. Cancer of the skin.

118. Carcinoma of the bladder.

119. Tumour of the liver.

120. Bronchial carcinoma.

121. Nasal cancer.

a. Aromatic amines.
b. Vinyl chloride monomer.
c. Pitch, cutting oils and ultra-violet light.
d. Leather workers, hardwoods and nickel.
e. Uranium, nickel carbonyl, chromates and asbestos.

Occupational cancers

115. a. True
b. False There is usually a long latent period between time of first exposure and the appearance of the tumour.
c. True Due to the appearance of tumours at an earlier age than would normally be expected. However some tumours of occupational origin may have a very long latent period, e.g. asbestos related tumours and in these cases death may be after retirement age.
d. True May get an unusually large incidence of a tumour in a particular location related to an exposure in that area.
e. False The exposure does not need to be continuous.

116. a. False It is thought to be a multi-step process. Classically initiation, promotion and progression.
b. True These are known as oncogenes.
c. False Organotrophy is the term used to describe the induction of tumours at specific sites by chemical carcinogens.
d. False Chemicals are the group most associated.
e. True Used to evaluate the carcinogenic potential of chemicals by looking for a mutagenic effect in bacteria.

117. c. Sunlight is important to those who work regularly outdoors such as roadworkers and farmers. Also ionizing radiation.

118. a. Examples are Benzidine and MOCA. Chemical, dyestuff, rubber cable industries.

119. b. VCM is associated with angiosarcoma of the liver.

120. e. Also arsenic trioxide and arsenites found in smelting and pesticides. There is an increased risk of lung cancer in asbestos exposed workers who smoke.

121. d. A rare adenocarcinoma. The very fine dust produced by power tools on hardwoods is particularly carcinogenic.

Occupational cancers

122. Occupations recognized as having a carcinogenic risk:
  a. Road work.
  b. Shipbuilding.
  c. Hairdressing.
  d. Cabinet making.
  e. Drug manufacture.

123. With regard to the relationship between occupation and leukaemia the following are correct:
  a. Associated primarily with radium salts.
  b. Found in some cases of benzene exposure.
  c. Associated with the asbestos industry.
  d. Linked with ionizing radiation exposure.
  e. The rubber industry has been implicated.

124. With regard to mesothelioma the following are true:
  a. It is a secondary tumour of peritoneum and pleura.
  b. Most cases in UK are related to asbestos exposure.
  c. Was formerly a prescribed industrial disease.
  d. Smoking produces a higher incidence.
  e. Has a latent period of fifteen to twenty-five years.

Occupational cancers

122. a. True — Skin cancer due to ultra-violet light exposure. Also seamen and farmers.
    b. True — As complications of exposure to asbestos – lung cancer and mesothelioma.
    c. False — No specific recognized association.
    d. True — Cancer of nasal sinuses due to wood dust.
    e. True — Pharmaceutical manufacture of cytotoxic drugs potentially causing bone marrow tumours.

123. a. False — Radium salts are most associated with osteosarcoma in workers using luminous paints.
    b. True — Frequently as the end point of aplastic anaemia. The myeloid type is commonest.
    c. False
    d. True — Dose related relationship.
    e. True — Acute lymphoid leukaemia. Aetiology unknown.

124. a. False — It is a primary tumour.
    b. True
    c False — It still is.
    d. False — Smoking does not appear to be a contributory factor. It seems to increase the chances of those exposed to asbestos developing lung cancer.
    e. False — Latent period usually forty or more years.

Ergonomics

125. **Ergonomics:**
    a. Aims to optimize working conditions for its human operators.
    b. Makes use of anthropometrics.
    c. Tries to fit the person to the task.
    d. Concentrates largely on equipment design.
    e. Has a role in setting patterns of work.

126. **Musculoskeletal problems at work may be due to:**
    a. Excessive range, frequency and force of movement.
    b. Abnormal positioning of limbs or body.
    c. Primarily psychological factors.
    d. Static loading.
    e. Lack of motivation.

127. **Factors contributing to work related upper limb disorders (WRULDs) include:**
    a. Poor work design – task factors.
    b. Environmental factors – such as task lighting and temperature.
    c. Inadequate protective equipment.
    d. Sudden or prolonged increases in work rates.
    e. Inadequate pre-employment assessment.

128. **The following are all clinical entities commonly associated with WRULDs:**
    a. Tenosynovitis.
    b. Ganglion.
    c. Carpal tunnel syndrome.
    d. Tendonitis crepitans.
    e. Acromioclavicular dislocation.

129. **Features of WRULDs are:**
    a. Inflammation of tendon or tendon sheaths.
    b. Diagnosis is usually obvious.
    c. Finger tip ulceration due to ischaemia.
    d. Relationship with prolonged static postures.
    e. Dominant hand more often affected.

125.
a. True — Fitting the task to the person.
b. True — This is the use of measurements relating to height, shoulder width, reach, arm span, etc. and body movements.
c. False — The task to the person.
d. False — The environment, the individual and the work design are also taken into account.
e. True

126.
a. True
b. True
c. False — Psychological factors (such as stress) may have a bearing but not necessarily a primary role.
d. True
e. False — May contribute to a greater or lesser extent but unlikely to be the sole cause of a musculoskeletal disorder.

127.
a. True
b. True
c. False — Only if the PPE contributes to poor work design.
d. True
e. False — Pre-employment assessment will not identify those likely to suffer from WRULDs except if a past history is elicited.

128.
a. True
b. False
c. True — Also radial and cubital tunnel syndrome.
d. True — Also epicondylitis and de Quervain's disorder.
e. False

129.
a. True — Or trauma of these structures.
b. False — Diagnosis is difficult.
c. False — This is a feature of hand-arm-vibration syndrome.
d. True — Also awkward and extremes of posture.
e. True

Ergonomics

130. In the carpal tunnel syndrome:
   a. Hyperaesthesia is restricted to the median nerve distribution.
   b. Wrist extension for one minute causes tingling in fingers (Phalen's test).
   c. There is an association with acromegaly.
   d. Tinel's test may be positive.
   e. Forceful, repetitive movements can cause median nerve neuropathy.

131. In tenosynovitis:
   a. The principal lesion is inflammation of a tendon.
   b. Excessive unaccustomed exercise may be causative.
   c. There are no apparent X-ray changes.
   d. Gentle exercise may give symptomatic relief.
   e. Work-related cases are bilateral.

Ergonomics

130. a. True
 b. False Phalen's test is wrist flexion for one minute producing tingling in the fingers.
 c. True Also myxoedema and fluid retention in pregnancy.
 d. True This is tingling in fingers produced by percussion over the carpal tunnel.
 e. True Due to both mechanical and ischaemic mechanisms.

131. a. False This is tendonitis. Tenosynovitis involves inflammation of the lining of the tendon sheath.
 b. True As well as repetitive microtrauma and strain.
 c. False Calcification in the tendon sheath may on occasion be found.
 d. False Relief is usually provided by rest or immobilization of the part.
 e. False Can be either unilateral or bilateral depending on nature of the work.

Microbiological hazards

Match the following (food poisoning):

132. Salmonella food poisoning.

133. *Staph. aureus* food poisoning.

134. *Clostridium welchii* food poisoning.

135. *Bacillus cerus* food poisoning.

136. *Clostridium botulinum* food poisoning.
  a. Toxin. Spore producing organism. Onset of symptoms one to sixteen hours. Associated with fried rice.
  b. Toxin. Can be rapidly fatal. Onset of symptoms within eighteen to thirty-six hours.
  c. Onset of symptoms in two to six hours. Organism found in skin folds, nasal passages and septic skin lesions.
  d. Onset of symptoms in two to seventy-two hours. Biggest single cause of food poisoning in UK. Associated with poultry and poultry products.
  e. Enterotoxin – onset of symptoms in eight to twenty-four hours. Anaerobic organism.

Microbiological hazards

132. d. Most common strain is *S. typhimurium*.

133. c. A toxin is produced by the bacterium. Recovery is rapid (within six hours).

134. e. Found in human and animal excreta as well as on raw meat. Illness may last one to three days.

135. a.

136. b. Rare in the UK. Anaerobic spore-producing bacterium which produces a potent toxin.

Microbiological hazards

Match the following (food hygiene):

137. Conditions for bacterial growth.

138. Risk factors when controlling contamination.

139. Assessment of food handlers.

140. Action following outbreak of food poisoning.

141. Ideal factory or kitchen environments.
   a. Condition of raw food and hygiene of handlers. Cleanliness of kitchens and equipment. Conditions for food storage.
   b. Exclude infectious diseases. Investigate diarrhoeal illness. Disqualify active and persistent infective discharges from ears, nose and eyes.
   c. Notify Public Health Department, identify affected persons and source for analysis. Share information with EHO, local hospitals, laboratories and GPs.
   d. Clean premises/machinery with adequate ventilation and waste disposal. Separate cloakroom facilities. Maintained refrigerators/chillers for food storage.
   e. Suitable food medium and temperature. Adequate moisture and sufficient time.

NOTE: EHO = Environment Health Officer

142. **With regard to microbiological hazards:**
   a. There are six bacterial diseases in the schedule of prescribed diseases.
   b. Human immunodeficiency virus (HIV) is a prescribed disease.
   c. Ankylostomiasis is the only helminthic disease in the schedule of prescribed diseases.
   d. Anyone contracting one of the prescribed microbiological diseases is entitled to compensation.
   e. Occupations most at risk include laboratory workers, health care workers and animal handlers.

Microbiological hazards

137. e. In general bacteria do not multiply below 15°C and above 40°C. Spores will be killed only at high temperatures such as boiling.

138. a. Most food poisoning outbreaks are the result of poor food handler hygiene.

139. b.

140. c. Non-return to work by those infected until shown to be clear of infection (stool sampling).

141. d. Also trained and informed staff. Good hygienic systems of work are important.

142. a. True   Anthrax, glanders, leptospirosis, tuberculosis, farmers' lung, brucella abortus.
    b. False   Viral hepatitis as the result of an occupation involving contact with human blood or blood products or contact with a source of viral hepatitis is the only viral disease in the list of prescribed diseases.
    c. True   Rare in the UK. Associated with work in or around mines.
    d. False   Contraction of the disease must be in the context of satisfying the occupational requirement as laid down in the schedule of prescribed diseases.
    e. True

Microbiological hazards

143. **Lyme disease**
   a. Was first recognized in Australia.
   b. Is caused by infectious spores entering the body.
   c. Is characterized by erythema multiforme.
   d. Has sheep and cattle as the primary animal reservoir in the UK.
   e. May be associated with neurological symptoms following infection.

144. **The following statements with regard to leptospirosis are correct:**
   a. When caused by bacterium *L. icterohaemorrhagiae* is known as Weil's disease.
   b. Primary preventive measure is drainage of wet ground.
   c. Is a prescribed industrial disease.
   d. Vaccination is available to workers at risk in the UK.
   e. Is not a serious illness and symptoms subside quickly.

145. **With regard to hepatitis B (HBV) the following are correct:**
   a. Health care workers are particularly at risk.
   b. Vaccination for HBV is 100 per cent effective.
   c. There is a recognized risk of transmission in mouth-to-mouth resuscitation manoeuvres in first aid.
   d. Surgeons who remain HBV antigen positive despite vaccination are medically retired.
   e. No risk of infection following a bite by a known carrier.

146. **In hepatitis B (HBV):**
   a. A major prolongation of prothrombin time is common.
   b. Incubation period is six to twenty-five weeks.
   c. Chronicity occurs in over 50 per cent of cases.
   d. Presence of HbsAg (surface antigen) indicates acute infection.
   e. There is no association with hepatocelluar carcinoma.

143.
a. False — Lyme, Connecticut, USA. It is an occupational zoonosis, i.e. an infectious disease transmitted from animals to man and contracted in the course of employment.
b. False — Is caused by bacterium *Borrelia burgdorferri* which is transmitted by the tick *Ixodes ricinus*.
c. False — It is erythema chronicum migrans – an area of redness spreading out from the site of the bite.
d. False — Usually associated with deer.
e. True — Facial nerve neuritis, myelitis, encephalitis and meningitis may all occur as may a myocarditis. Chronic polyarthritis may also be found.

144.
a. True — Is an occupational zoonosis.
b. False — It is the control of rats whose urine contains the bacteria.
c. True
d. False
e. False — It is a serious disease with up to 20 per cent of cases being fatal.

145.
a. True — For example, during surgical procedures and needlestick injuries.
b. False — Sero-conversion is 80–90 per cent.
c. False — There are no documented cases of transmission during this activity.
d. False — They cannot do invasive work and need to be redeployed/retrained.
e. False — Can be transmitted by injury or being bitten by an infectious patient.

146.
a. False — It is uncommon and when present indicates severe illness.
b. True
c. False — In 5–10 per cent of cases.
d. True — Usually appears during incubation period. Is used to diagnose HBV.
e. False — Is associated with hepatocellular carcinoma, chronic hepatitis and cirrhosis.

Microbiological hazards

147. The following statements relating to hepatitis A (HAV) are correct:
  a. Incubation period is eight to twelve weeks.
  b. Sewerage workers may be at risk.
  c. A vaccine is not available.
  d. Most infections are subclinical.
  e. Chronic carrier states are common.

148. Features of hepatitis C (HCV):
  a. Common in children and young adults.
  b. Transmitted in blood and blood products.
  c. Average incubation period of two to four weeks.
  d. May be transmitted in a needlestick injury.
  e. Vaccination is available for health care workers.

149. In acquired immune deficiency syndrome (AIDS):
  a. Risk of infection from needlestick injury is greater than for HBV.
  b. There is an association with chlamydia pneumoniae.
  c. Workplace infection risk is low.
  d. A transmissible retrovirus is the causative agent.
  e. Full informed consent is required before HIV testing is performed.

Match the following:

150. Anthrax (*B. anthracis*).
151. Leptospirosis.
152. Brucellosis (*B. abortus*).
153. Hepatitis B (HBV).
154. Legionellosis (*L. pneumophilia*).

  a. Contracted from infected bovine carcasses or ingesting raw milk.
  b. Occurs in outbreaks. Associated with cooling towers and air conditioning systems.
  c. From infected blood or blood products. Needlestick injury an important occupational factor.
  d. Handling of wool, hides and carcases of infected animals. Two forms: cutaneous and pulmonary.
  e. Flu-like illness with jaundice. Involves contact with urine of rodents, dogs or bovines.

Microbiological hazards

147. a. False   Two to six weeks.
     b. True
     c. False   Hepatitis A vaccine is available.
     d. True   And thus unrecognized.
     e. False   HAV has no known carrier state and plays no role in the production of chronic active hepatitis or cirrhosis.

148. a. False   Tends to be associated with post-transfusion hepatitis and contaminated needle sharing in drug misusers.
     b. True
     c. False   It is seven to eight weeks.
     d. True
     e. False   Vaccine against HCV has not yet been developed.

149. a. False   Estimated to be less of a risk.
     b. False   Associated with *Pneumocystis carinii* pneumonia.
     c. True   HIV has extremely low risk of transmission by casual contact and accidental infection is rare. However some workers may be exposed to the possibility of needlestick injuries and contamination of broken skin or mucous membranes, e.g. health care workers, prison or police officers.
     d. True
     e. True

150. d. Rare in the UK. Imported bone/fish meal account for most cases. Hides, wool and hair from the Far and Middle East have potential to transmit the infection.

151. e. Occupations at risk include farmers, sewerage and watercourse workers.

152. a. Rare in the UK. Occupational contraction is usually by handling infected animals (placental or fetal tissue in particular) or by inhalation of infected aerosols from such animals.

153. c.

154. b. Causes an atypical pneumonia.

Mental health

155. **With regard to mental health at work:**
     a. Physical well-being is not important.
     b. Equilibrium between work and home environments is important.
     c. Influenced by an individual's personality and culture.
     d. Genetic predisposition important.
     e. Occupational issues alone may cause problems.

156. **The following statements relating to stress at work are correct:**
     a. May be related to poor job satisfaction.
     b. Individuals likely to suffer can be identified at the pre-employment stage.
     c. Underwork is less important than overwork.
     d. Minimized by personnel policies that promote individual self-respect, personal development and feelings of worth.
     e. Commonly related to clinical entities of neuroses and psychoses.

157. **In occupational stress:**
     a. Prolonged overwork under pressure can lead to mental and physical health problems.
     b. A stressed employee may typically experience hallucinations and exhibit delusional thoughts.
     c. Some individuals are susceptible whilst others are not.
     d. Drug and alcohol abuse frequently lead to its development.
     e. The role of the manager is most important.

155. a. False
b. True
c. True
d. False — May be a factor in the work setting for some individuals but not generally important.
e. True — Work-related issues can themselves cause mental health problems.

156. a. True
b. False — Not always the case.
c. False — Both are important factors.
d. True
e. False — These may be present in some individuals but overall they are not common causes of work-related stress. However forms of neurosis may develop secondary to the original work-related stress.

157. a. True
b. False — These are psychotic symptoms. The stressed employee may show lack of concentration, poor time-keeping/productivity, apathy, irritability and resentment.
c. True — Individual personality and ability to cope varies. Hence what may be stress to one individual may be a challenge to another – the early identification of the loss of an individual's capacity to cope is important in the management of stress.
d. False — It is more likely that feelings of stress at work may lead some individuals to abuse alcohol or drugs.
e. True — Firstly, they must be aware of the signs of stress and secondly they should communicate well with employees, provide encouragement and support and ensure training to carry out the job is adequate.

Mental health

158. Stress management:
  a. Should take account of the different abilities individuals have to withstand stressors at work.
  b. Requires that direct supervisors have a limited role.
  c. In the workplace involves separating out non-work stressors and dealing only with those related to the occupation.
  d. Encourages the development of coping strategies within the workplace.
  e. May be helped by the presence of a workplace mental health policy.

159. Recognized features of depression are:
  a. Poor concentration and indecisiveness.
  b. Paranoid delusions.
  c. Psychomotor retardation and fatigue.
  d. Thought disorder.
  e. Suicidal ideation.

160. The following statements relating to shift work are correct:
  a. Sleep difficulties are experienced by those on night shifts.
  b. Standardized mortality ratios (SMRs) for night workers are higher than for those on day shift.
  c. Health problems affect women significantly more than men.
  d. Insulin dependent diabetics should not work on night shifts.
  e. Younger age groups cope better with shift work.

Mental health

158. a. True Reaction to stressors highlights individual variability.
b. False They have a key role to be aware of and recognize problems at an early stage.
c. False It may be difficult to deal with outside stressors, e.g. domestic disharmony, however their importance cannot be ignored.
d. True Mechanisms to help individuals cope with stress should be developed.
e. True Such a policy must be comprehensive, cover agreed objectives and be consistently applied.

159. a. True
b. False
c. True
d. False This is a characteristic feature of schizophrenia.
e. True

160. a. True Particularly if there is rapid alternation between spells on day and night shifts.
b. False SMRs are virtually the same for both categories.
c. False
d. False In particular the advent of multi-dose insulin regimes are useful in allowing diabetics to participate in shift work.
e. True

Medical examinations

161. With regard to the occupational history the following are true:
   a. Deals only with the effect of work on health.
   b. Hobbies and pastime activities should be included.
   c. Previous jobs are less important than the current job.
   d. Will always involve a detailed assessment of exposure to workplace hazards.
   e. Allows an assessment to be made on fitness to return to work after illness or injury.

162. Investigation of occupational disease will involve:
   a. The use of epidemiological tools.
   b. The assessment of crude occupational mortality statistics to provide an accurate reference source of occupation and mortality.
   c. Using the job title as a good indicator of occupational exposure.
   d. The important use of clinical observation coupled with an occupational history.
   e. Disease registers.

163. Rehabilitation includes the following:
   a. The process by which people with disabilities are helped to return to work.
   b. Medical rehabilitation preceeding occupational rehabilitation.
   c. Activities that help an individual return to former employment or be redeployed with new skills.
   d. Assessment of disability and employment handicap as the most important aspect.
   e. Employment rehabilitation centres which are involved in assessment, employment rehabilitation and job-seek training.

Medical examinations

161. a. False   The practice of occupational medicine is based on the concept of the effect of work on health and the effect of health on work.
    b. True   These may be relevant, e.g. the use of adhesives for model making in a case of occupational asthma.
    c. False   Previous job history is important, particularly if dealing with chronic disease.
    d. False   Will be detailed only if a work-related disease is suspected. Then an in-depth history is needed of what the worker has been exposed to, for how long and in what quantities.
    e. True   Realistic and more accurate advice can be given to both employee and employers.

162. a. True
    b. False   Information may not be accurate due to bias in the description of the occupation, i.e. the deceased tends to get 'promoted' when the death is registered.
    c. False   Job title may not be specific enough to allow correlation with an occupational exposure.
    d. True
    e. True   These give ill-health specifically related to work, e.g. *SWORD* (*Surveillance of Work Related and Occupational Chest Diseases*) or *RIDDOR* (*Reporting of Injuries, Diseases and Dangerous Occurrences Regulations*).

163. a. True   After they have had some kind of illness or injury.
    b. False   Medical rehabilitation reduces the extent of any disability resulting from an impairment. Occupational rehabilitation reduces the extent of the employment handicap resulting from a disability. Both should proceed together where possible.
    c. False   That is resettlement.
    d. True   To allow a determination of functional recovery after injury/illness and hence whether a return to work/redeployment is feasible.
    e. True.

Medical examinations

164. In cases of back pain:
   a. Most are functional in origin.
   b. Sleeplessness at night indicates a mechanical origin.
   c. Where an injury has occurred there is an increased risk of recurrence.
   d. Acute disc prolapse may occur due to sudden back strain or awkward lifting posture.
   e. Job task design is important in prevention.

165. The following statements with regard to ill-health retirement are correct:
   a. It should be considered only when it is clear that an employee's health problem prevents a return to previous employment.
   b. An employer cannot dismiss an employee with a genuine health problem.
   c. The occupational physician may recommend it if the work environment would continually affect an employee's health adversely.
   d. The company medical officer is usually well placed to give advice.
   e. It is the occupational physician's duty to ensure that redeployment has been considered before proceeding with the recommendation.

166. Features of prolapsed intervertebral disc are:
   a. L3 or L4 nerve roots most often affected.
   b. S1 radiculopathy causes loss of ankle jerk.
   c. L5 nerve root compression results in extensor plantar response.
   d. Retention of urine.
   e. Pain made worse by Valsalva manoeuvre.

167. In vocational driving (LGV and PCV):
   a. A higher fitness standard is required than for ordinary driving.
   b. A myocardial infarction is a bar to vocational driving.
   c. Drivers with epilepsy are barred from vocational driving.
   d. Insulin dependent diabetes is a prescribed disability under road traffic legislation.
   e. Minimum vision standard for new applicants is 6/9 and 6/12 corrected.

Medical examinations

164.
a. False — Most cases are mechanical in origin.
b. False — Back pain causing sleeplessness should be considered to be serious and malignancy must be ruled out. Mechanical back pain may cause difficulty getting to sleep or waking due to movement causing pain.
c. True — Particularly with prolapsed intervertrebral disc lesions.
d. True — There is back pain, sciatica (L5,S1), reduced spinal movements and straight leg raising. Neurological signs may be present.
e. True

165.
a. True — But relocation may still be an option.
b. False — If the employee is unsatisfactory the cause may not be important. However established disciplinary procedures must have been followed. Retirement on ill-health grounds could be an alternative option.
c. True
d. True — They will know the task and thus the requirements in terms of fitness for the job.
e. True

166.
a. False — Most often affects L5 or S1 nerve roots.
b. True — Also sensory loss over lateral calf and foot.
c. False — There is foot drop and sensory loss over shin and dorsum of foot.
d. True — Due to cauda equina compression – urgent referral required.
e. True — For example coughing, laughing, straining at stool.

167.
a. True
b. False — Provided satisfactory recovery is made, there is no angina and treadmill test satisfies the guidelines of the Secretary of State's Honorary Medical Advisory Panel, vocational driving may be allowed subject to medical assessment.
c. False — If seizure-free for ten years, on no treatment during that time, and the liability to seizure is deemed to be low – these cases may drive vocationally subject to medical assessment.
d. True
e. True — And 3/60 uncorrected.

Medical examinations

168. With regard to occupational disease the following are correct:
   a. Angiosarcoma of the liver in vinyl chloride workers is increasing.
   b. Information from Registrar of Deaths gives good occupational data.
   c. Occupational metal poisoning has declined in the developed world.
   d. *Reporting of Injuries, Diseases and Dangerous Occurrences Regulations* (*RIDDOR*) shows a tendency to under reporting.
   e. Environmental factors can be relevant in determining health.

169. The following statements relating to pre-employment medical examinations are correct:
   a. It is the best way of determining fitness for work.
   b. Replacement by questionnaire assessment may miss vital information.
   c. They are statutory for some types of jobs, e.g. divers and those working with ionizing radiation.
   d. Clinical information cannot be disclosed without the written informed consent of the examinee.
   e. Can be useful in obtaining base-line data.

170. Disabled workers:
   a. Have a higher than average rate of absence.
   b. Restrictions (if any) placed on them should be appropriate and precise.
   c. Were provided with enhanced employment opportunities by the disabled quota scheme.
   d. Represent an increased safety risk in the workplace.
   e. Will achieve limited benefit from the occupational health team.

168. a. False   May have appeared in clusters but is declining due to control measures.
      b. False   It is open to incorrect or vague diagnosis of cause of death and a tendency for relatives to misreport the occupation.
      c. True
      d. True   Employers have the responsibility of reporting to HSE certain accidents and diseases.
      e. True   Particularly the work environment when so much of a person's life is spent at work.

169. a. False   It is important to determine the psychological and physical requirements for a job and apply the best/most cost effective means of detecting those who would not be suitable. It is important that the criteria applied are appropriate and not overly restrictive without good reason.
      b. False
      c. True   Also lead workers.
      d. True   Medical confidentiality is most important at all times in the occupational health setting and not just at pre-employment examinations.
      e. True   An example would be base-line audiograms for those working in a noisy environment.

170. a. False   Many will be highly motivated to overcome their disability and hence attendance rates may be better than average.
      b. True   Restrictions should have a good reason for being imposed and be based on sound health or safety grounds.
      c. False   The quota system (employers of 20 or more employees must have a workforce with 3 per cent registered disabled persons) was very poorly complied with.
      d. False   Provided they are correctly placed there is no increased safety risk.
      e. False   The occupational health team can give advice to an employer on modifications needed to allow a disabled employee to be employed or remain in employment if the disability is progressive.

Medical examinations

171. With regard to sickness absence the following are correct:
   a. It is any absence from work attributed to incapacity.
   b. Can be measured in a variety of ways including percentage of time lost and average length of spells.
   c. Young people tend to take more uncertified absence than the older worker.
   d. Genuine medical illness exists in most cases.
   e. Past attendance record has no bearing in a new job.

172. In the control of sickness absence:
   a. Pre-employment medicals are good predictors.
   b. Management readily accepts responsibility for control.
   c. A comprehensive written policy on sickness absence is useful in dealing with this issue.
   d. Keeping staff informed on their levels of absence is worthwhile.
   e. The International Labour Organisation endorse an occupational physician being asked to justify another physician's incapacity certificate.

173. The following statements with regard to alcohol problems in the workplace are correct:
   a. May be indicated by a pattern of Monday absenteeism and deteriorating work performance.
   b. The occupational health team should be involved in all aspects of a disciplinary policy including taking samples of blood or urine.
   c. An alcohol policy should be agreed by all including top management.
   d. Alcohol abuse in the workplace should, in the interests of the problem drinker, not be treated in confidence.
   e. The rules and penalties governing problem drinking must be clearly stated in an alcohol policy.

Medical examinations

171.
- a. True
- b. True
- c. True — Although certified sickness absence increases with increasing age.
- d. False — In many cases there may be no genuine medical illness present.
- e. False — Past attendance is the best predictor for future attendance.

172.
- a. False — Past attendance record is best indicator.
- b. False — Surprisingly not in all organizations.
- c. True
- d. True
- e. False — The opposite is true.

173.
- a. True — Also poor time-keeping, increased accident rates, abusive behaviour and overt smell of alcohol on breath at work.
- b. False — The role of the occupational health team should be divorced from the mechanics of any disciplinary procedures such as these.
- c. True — This is vital.
- d. False — Medical confidentiality guidelines must apply in all cases.
- e. True

Medical examinations

174. Drug abuse:
a. Outside the workplace is unlikely to affect work performance.
b. May cause the following to be exhibited: behavioural changes, irritability, mood swings, impaired work performance and poor time-keeping.
c. Is controlled in the UK by the *Misuse of Drugs Act 1971*.
d. Should be tackled in the workplace by having a policy on drug abuse as part of a comprehensive health and safety policy.
e. Involves the routine screening of those working in jobs involving responsibility for the safety of others, e.g. pilots, train drivers.

175. Considerations in workplace health promotion are:
a. It should form part of a comprehensive occupational health service.
b. A needs assessment should be the first step.
c. It can link in with the UK Government health strategy 'The Health of the Nation'.
d. Effectiveness has been scientifically proven.
e. Must have the support of management and the workforce.

176. Working in confined spaces:
a. Includes tanks, culverts, tunnels and trenches.
b. May lead to some medical restrictions being imposed such as epilepsy, angina and vertigo.
c. Has lack of room to manoeuvre as the main hazard.
d. Can be carried out if it is well ventilated before entry.
e. May require routine health surveillance of workers as a good practice.

177. Consideration of reproductive health in the workplace will include the following:
a. VDU work is commonly associated with miscarriage.
b. Reproductive hazards in the occupational environment are rare.
c. Physically strenuous work activity in females may lead to amenorrhoea.
d. In most cases of fetal abnormality the cause is unknown.
e. Toxic substances can exert an effect at any stage in the reproductive cycle.

Medical examinations

174.
- a. False — It may do so.
- b. True — Remember other causes of these signs, e.g. alcohol abuse or anxiety.
- c. True — It covers nearly all drugs with abuse/dependance properties.
- d. True — It should aim to minimize or eradicate the effect of drug abuse on the abuser, work colleagues and his work performance.
- e. False — Such screening is carried out but is not routine in the UK.

175.
- a. True
- b. True
- c. True — And those for the other UK regions.
- d. False — Outcomes are difficult to measure and hence evidence of effectiveness (outside the USA) is limited.
- e. True — Imposed health promotion programmes in the workplace may be ineffective.

176.
- a. True
- b. True — Also black-outs, fainting attacks, claustrophobia, visual defects and severe respiratory disease or exertional dyspnoea.
- c. False — The main problems arise due to oxygen deficiency or build up of toxic gases and subsequent asphyxia (e.g. CO_2, CO, methane and H_2S).
- d. True — Or if not feasible then appropriate breathing apparatus should be worn.
- e. True — This could be carried out by questionnaire in an attempt to identify any contraindicated medical condition.

177.
- a. False — There has been no epidemiological evidence to firmly link VDU work with any adverse pregnancy outcome.
- b. True
- c. True — Similar to that found in some female athletes.
- d. True — It has been suggested that 5 per cent are due to environmental factors of which none are directly related to occupation.
- e. True — This includes males and females. Effects may be infertility, loss of libido, miscarriage and fetal abnormality.

Medical examinations

178. Features of sick building syndrome are:
 a. Lethargy and tiredness.
 b. Equal sex distribution.
 c. Migraine headaches.
 d. Influenza-like symptoms.
 e. Association with air conditioning systems.

179. Iron deficiency anaemia has the following features:
 a. Low serum ferritin.
 b. Total iron binding capacity is low.
 c. MCV is reduced.
 d. Reticulocytopaenia.
 e. Normal erythrocyte count.

180. The following are recognized causes of finger clubbing:
 a. Bronchial carcinoma.
 b. Legionellosis.
 c. Hepatic cirrhosis.
 d. Tuberculosis.
 e. Bacterial endocarditis.

181. The following are associated with Parkinsonism:
 a. Bradykinesia.
 b. Carbon monoxide poisoning.
 c. Difficulty performing repetitive type work.
 d. Hypotonia.
 e. Torticollis.

182. Considering epilepsy and work:
 a. Those with the condition are more likely to be unemployed.
 b. Photosensitivity is a common feature affecting choice of work.
 c. Higher than average accident rate.
 d. Exclusion from work with VDUs.
 e. Work performance is equivalent to or better than the average.

183. The pregnant worker:
 a. Is suspended from work with lead.
 b. Cannot be dismissed for pregnancy-related reasons.
 c. Should avoid working with VDUs.
 d. Is entitled to fourteen weeks' maternity leave dependent on years of service.
 e. Can retain a company car during maternity leave.

Medical examinations

178.
a. True
b. False — More females appear to suffer than males.
c. False — Headaches are common but migraine is not a typical feature of them.
d. True
e. True — Seems to be more apparent when compared with naturally ventilated buildings.

179.
a. True — As is serum iron level.
b. False — It is high.
c. True — MCH is also reduced.
d. True
e. False

180.
a. True
b. False
c. True
d. False
e. True

181.
a. True — Slowing of movements.
b. True — Is a cause of secondary Parkinsonism.
c. True — Slowness, rigidity and tremor may affect ability to perform repetitive type work.
d. False
e. False

182.
a. True
b. False — It is rare.
c. False — Similar to the average.
d. False — Only those with photosensitive epilepsy should not.
e. True — As is sickness absence.

183.
a. True
b. True — To do so may be an unfair dismissal.
c. False
d. False — Entitlement is regardless of length of service or hours worked – *Trade Union Reform and Employment Rights Act 1993 (TURERA)*.
e. True — A woman's contractual terms must be continued during maternity leave (*TURERA*). If she had use of a company car prior to pregnancy she could be entitled to continued use.

General toxicology

Match the following:

184. Vapours.
185. Fumes
186. Mists
187. Aerosols

a. Solid particles generated by condensation from the gaseous state, generally after volatization from molten metals.
b. Liquid droplets or solid particles dispersed in air of a fine enough particle size to remain dispersed for some time.
c. Gaseous form of a substance normally solid or liquid which occurs by the process of evaporation.
d. Suspended droplets generated by condensation from gaseous to liquid state or the breaking up of a liquid into a dispersed state.

188. **In toxicology:**
   a. Inhalation is a less important route of entry for a toxic substance than percutaneous absorption.
   b. There can be individual susceptibility in reaction to exposure of a toxic substance.
   c. Metabolism of a non-toxic substance may provide a toxic metabolite.
   d. Possible toxic effects include irritation, allergy and asphyxiation.
   e. Latent periods can be associated with most toxic substances.

189. **In metal toxicology:**
   a. Metal absorption into the body is most effective via the gut.
   b. Some metals undergo biotransformation.
   c. Age is an important factor in metal poisoning.
   d. Dietary considerations are unimportant.
   e. Important factors relating to toxicity are particle size, solubility and interactions between metals.

190. **Biological monitoring:**
   a. Is applicable to substances that act locally.
   b. Can be used to detect peak exposures to rapidly acting substances.
   c. Gives a biological index of internal dose.
   d. Takes account of all routes of absorption.
   e. Involves measurement of the agent or its metabolite usually in the blood or urine.

General toxicology

184. c. Occur by the process of evaporation at a solid or liquid surface.

185. a. The change is often associated with a chemical change, e.g. oxidation. Fume particles may be very fine, i.e. less than 1 μm.

186. d. May form as the result of splashing, atomizing or foaming. Examples are mists from cutting/grinding oils.

187. b.

188.
- a. False — Inhalation would be the principal route of entry for many toxic substances in the occupational setting.
- b. True
- c. True — The converse is also true.
- d. True
- e. False

189.
- a. False — Generally absorption is more effective via the lungs than the gut.
- b. False — No metals are bio-transformed, most are excreted in urine.
- c. True — In general as age increases the absorption of metals from the gut decreases.
- d. False — Constituents of diet may cause interactions, e.g. lead absorption varies inversely with calcium and iron in diet.
- e. True — Particle size is important for lung absorption, i.e. they must be respirable. Interactions between metals will influence uptake as will solubility.

190.
- a. False — Not usually applicable to locally acting substances or in detecting peak exposures to rapidly acting substances.
- b. False
- c. True — This is likely to be more closely related to a systemic effect than any environmental measurement.
- d. True — And individual variation.
- e. True — It is the measurement and assessment of workplace agents or their metabolites either in tissues, secreta, excreta or any combination of these to evaluate exposure and health risk compared with an appropriate reference standard.

General toxicology

191. In carbon monoxide poisoning:
a. There is cyanotic skin discolouration.
b. Hyperbaric oxygen therapy may be used in treatment.
c. Industrial exposure is a common source.
d. Death usually occurs with 60–80 per cent carboxyhaemoglobin.
e. Fifty per cent oxygen is used in immediate treatment.

192. With regard to lead the following are correct:
a. The suspension level for lead in blood of male workers is 70 μg/dl (3.5 μmol/l).
b. Suspension is required when blood lead is greater than 30 μg/dl (1.5 μmol/l) in women of child-bearing age.
c. Lead poisoning is one of the commonest forms of occupational poisoning in the UK.
d. Inorganic lead is absorbed through the skin.
e. In occupational lead exposure inhalation is the main route of entry.

193. In relation to mercury the following statements are true:
a. Poisoning by mercury or a mercury compound is a prescribed disease.
b. Elemental, alkyl and inorganic forms are the most toxic.
c. Mercury workers usually have blood mercury levels periodically monitored.
d. Principal target organs are the kidney and central nervous system.
e. Acute poisoning is common from occupational exposure and is usually due to ingestion.

194. With regard to cadmium (Cd) the following are true:
a. Acute effects of cadmium poisoning after inhalation of fumes may show a delay in presentation.
b. Chronic poisoning principally affects the liver.
c. May get discolouration in teeth.
d. Is linked to high risk of prostatic cancer.
e. Biological monitoring of exposed workers involves both blood and urinary estimations.

General toxicology

191. a. False   It is cherry-red.
    b. True
    c. True   For example exhaust gases and afterdamp in mines.
    d. True
    e. False   100 per cent oxygen or 95 per cent oxygen with 5 per cent carbon dioxide.

192. a. True
    b. False   Suspension for women of child-bearing age is 40 μg/dl (2.0 μmol/l). 70 μg/dl (3.5 μmol/l) is correct for males. *Lead at Work Regulations (1980)* and *Revised Code of Practice (1985)*.
    c. False   This is true for developing countries however.
    d. False   Organo-leads may be absorbed through the skin (tetraethyl lead).
    e. True   Although ingestion remains important especially if personal hygiene is poor leading to contamination of ingested food.

193. a. True
    b. True
    c. False   It is (in UK) the periodic measurement of mercury in urine.
    d. True   Inorganic mercury does not cross blood–brain barrier as readily as elemental or alkyl forms.
    e. False   Acute poisoning is not common in an occupational setting. When it does occur it is usually as a result of inhalation of mercury vapour.

194. a. True   Acute effects due to inhalation of Cd oxide fumes may show a latent period of up to ten hours – chest pain, dyspnoea and cough.
    b. False   The kidney: tubular damage.
    c. True   Yellowing of teeth may occur in Cd poisoning.
    d. False   The risk, if it is present at all, is small.
    e. True

General toxicology

195. The following statements relating to arsenic are correct:
 a. Occupational exposure is likely to occur in pesticide/herbicide manufacture and smelting.
 b. Has a very short half-life in blood.
 c. Chronic poisoning may cause skin changes.
 d. Associated with angiosarcoma of liver.
 e. The characteristic respiratory tract lesion is cancer of maxillary sinuses.

196. With regard to manganese (Mn) the following are correct:
 a. Is well absorbed through the intestine and easily crosses the blood–brain barrier.
 b. Poisoning is characterized by two phases.
 c. Periodic medical examinations are useful.
 d. Uptake is associated with iron deficiency.
 e. An individual susceptibility to manganese poisoning is described.

197. In relation to phosphorous the following statements are true:
 a. Red phosphorous is usually associated with necrosis of the jaw.
 b. Poisoning is a prescribed disease.
 c. May cause serious burns on skin contact.
 d. Dental examinations are an important feature in monitoring.
 e. Phosphine gas is a hazard associated with the manufacture of pesticides.

General toxicology

195. a. True   Also in chemical and pharmaceutical industries.
      b. False   Half-life in blood is two to two-and-a-half days. It is rapidly eliminated via the kidney.
      c. True   Skin ulceration, hyperkeratosis of palms and soles. Hyperpigmentation and eczematous dermatitis. Also skin cancer.
      d. True   And lung cancer.
      e. False   It is perforation of nasal cartilaginous septum.

196. a. False   It is poorly absorbed from GIT and crosses blood–brain barrier with difficulty.
      b. False   Three phases: (i) general lassitude, tiredness, pains (ii) dysarthria, imbalance and hypersalivation (iii) Parkinsonian type features.
      c. True   To detect early behavioural or neurological changes.
      d. True   The uptake of Mn from the intestine is enhanced by a deficiency in iron.
      e. True   Due to an interaction with iron, those who have an increased GIT uptake of iron have an increased Mn uptake. Anaemic individuals absorb Mn at a higher level than normal.

197. a. False   Jaw necrosis is usually associated with white (or yellow) phosphorous – phossy jaw. Today white phosphorous is used in explosives/munitions manufacture. Incidence of jaw necrosis is extremely rare now compared with the end of last century/early twentieth century, when it was found in match makers.
      b. True
      c. True
      d. True
      e. False   A very toxic asphyxiant gas formed in the manufacture of acetylene.

General toxicology

198. With regard to beryllium the following are correct:
a. May get an allergic contact dermatitis.
b. GIT absorption is good.
c. Is associated with a chronic pulmonary condition.
d. Chronic poisoning is associated with gliomatous lesions.
e. Blood beryllium levels are a reliable method of biological monitoring.

199. The following statements in relation to glutaraldehyde are correct:
a. Has antimicrobial properties.
b. Health care workers are at risk of toxic effects.
c. Formic acid in urine is used to monitor exposure.
d. Is a known sensitizer.
e. Has teratogenic effects.

200. In relation to acrylamide the following are true:
a. Poisoning is associated with both polymer and monomer.
b. Acute effects are those of irritation to skin and mucus membranes.
c. Upper and lower limb paraesthesia is a complication of poisoning.
d. Inhalation is commonest route of entry.
e. Chronic poisoning is associated with mid-brain lesions.

201. Regarding vanadium the following statements are correct:
a. Inhalation is the principal route of entry.
b. Excessive exposure can be associated with metallic taste in mouth and a green/black tongue.
c. Main effects due to over exposure relate to irritation of mucus membranes.
d. Blood vanadium estimation is the preferred method of biological monitoring.
e. A coarse Parkinsonian type tremor.

198. a. True   Beryllium acts as a skin sensitizer.
     b. False   GIT absorption is poor. Lung absorption is rapid.
     c. True   Berylliosis or chronic beryllium disease.
     d. False   It is a sarcoid-like granulomatous lesion affecting lungs and also subcutaneous skin tissues.
     e. False   There are no reliable methods – beryllium can be found in urine of exposed workers, however, periodic chest X-rays and respiratory function tests are important in detecting early stages of Bc disease.

199. a. True   Hence its use as a sterilizing agent in endoscopy units.
     b. True   Principally nursing staff in endoscopy units.
     c. False   This is for formaldehyde, glutaraldehyde does not have any metabolite analogous to formic acid with which to monitor exposure.
     d. True   Can cause contact dermatitis and occupational asthma.
     e. False   Not shown to be the case in humans.

200. a. False   Only monomer is toxic.
     b. True   Blistering of skin may occur with prolonged contact.
     c. True   Peripheral neuropathy is a feature of chronic exposure usually of legs rather than arms.
     d. False   Skin absorption is the commonest route, lung and GIT absorption is possible but less common.
     e. True   Ataxia, tremor, dysarthria, increased sweating.

201. a. True
     b. True
     c. True   Respiratory tract irritation. Pneumonitis.
     d. False   Urinary vanadium estimation is the method recommended for assessment of exposure.
     e. False   A fine tremor of fingers and hands may be present in cases of toxicity.

General toxicology

202. With regard to chromium the following are true:
   a. Trivalent chromium salts are irritant, corrosive and carcinogenic.
   b. Chromium compounds are sensitizers.
   c. Is no longer a prescribed disease.
   d. Associated with nasal perforation.
   e. Urinary chromium measurement at the end of shifts is routinely used to measure exposure in workers.

Match the following:

203. Lead.   a. Urinary thiodyglycolic acid.

204. Trichloroethylene.   b. Urinary methyl hippuric acid.

205. Vinyl chloride monomer.   c. Urinary trichloroacetic acid.

206. Benzene.   d. Urinary ALA.

207. Xylene.   e. Urinary phenols.

208. The following are associated with causing cataract:
   a. Welding.
   b. Mercury poisoning.
   c. Electrocution.
   d. Beryllium.
   e. Dinitrophenol.

209. The following are known to cause peripheral neuropathy:
   a. Organophosphorus pesticides.
   b. Manganese.
   c. Vanadium pentoxide.
   d. Acrylamide.
   e. Thallium.

202. a. False   This describes hexavelant chromium salts where carcinogenicity is related to lung cancer. The trivalent salts are virtually non-toxic.
     b. True   Thus may cause contact dermatitis and occupational asthma.
     c. False   It is a prescribed disease for chronic irritation of skin and lung cancer from zinc chromate, calcium chromate or strontium chromate.
     d. True   Usually due to inhalation of chrome vapours, e.g. chrome plating tanks.
     e. False   Not routinely used in UK but is thought to give an index of recent exposure to soluble hexavelant chromium compounds.

203. d. Amino levalunic acid. Blood lead is used more frequently as a biological monitor.

204. c. Urinary metabolite used for biological monitoring.

205. a. Urinary metabolite used for biological monitoring.

206. e. Urinary metabolite used for biological monitoring.

207. b.

208. a. True   Due to infra-red radiation.
     b. False
     c. True   Rarely. May be a latent period of approximately one year before formation starts. Can resolve spontaneously.
     d. False   Causes a conjunctivitis.
     e. True

209. a. True
     b. False
     c. False
     d. True
     e. True

General toxicology

Match the following:

210. Lead poisoning.
211. Mercury poisoning.
212. Cadmium poisoning.
213. Chromium poisoning.
214. Manganese poisoning.

a. Brown-blue line on gums, fulminant itch, erethism, cerebellar cortical atrophy and dislocation of lens.
b. Skin ulceration, pneumonitis, asthma and lung cancer.
c. Respiratory irritation, organic psychosis and Parkinsonism.
d. Abdominal pain, anaemia, raised erythrocyte protoporphyrin and siderocytes in peripheral blood.
e. Focal emphysema, anosmia, renal calculi and glycosuria.

215. **In solvent toxicology:**
   a. Water soluble solvents penetrate the skin and accumulate in nervous tissues.
   b. All solvents in their vapour phase are rapidly absorbed through the lungs.
   c. Solvent volatility determines toxicity to an extent.
   d. All solvents are bio-transformed in the body and excreted as metabolites.
   e. Mixtures of solvents can cause biological competition and this interferes with the action of each component.

216. **Regarding chlorinated hydrocarbons the following are correct:**
   a. Are inflammable and explosive.
   b. Used widely as degreasing agents, paint solvents and dry-cleaning fluids.
   c. The introduction of the chlorine radicle decreases their toxicity.
   d. As molecular weight falls so does toxicity.
   e. Toxicity is related to volatility.

217. **The following statements relating to carbon disulphide are correct:**
   a. It is the most common organic chemical that contains a carbon sulphide group.
   b. Skin absorption is main route of entry.
   c. May be associated with infertility in males and females.
   d. Only recently widely used in the synthetic fibres industry.
   e. Is a recognized multi-system poison.

General toxicology

210. d. Also raised blood lead levels.

211. a. Erethism is a toxic organic psychosis.

212. e.

213. b.

214. c.

215. a. False This applies to lipid soluble solvents.
     b. True
     c. True The more volatile a solvent is the greater the possibility of it being in the atmosphere and hence being inhaled.
     d. False Not all are bio-transformed. Some are excreted unchanged in the urine.
     e. True

216. a. False They are non-inflammable, non-combustible and non-explosive hence their wide usage.
     b. True
     c. False The reverse is true.
     d. False The toxicity increases with increasing molecular weight.
     e. True

217. a. True
     b. False Skin absorption can occur but inhalation is primary route of entry.
     c. True
     d. False Has been in use for around 150 years. Originally used as a rubber solvent in 1850s.
     e. True Effects include peripheral neuropathy, ischaemic heart disease, psychosis and Parkinsonian effects.

General toxicology

218. Features of carbon tetrachloride are:
   a. A colourless, volatile and non-inflammable liquid with a sweet smelling odour.
   b. Water soluble solvent.
   c. A nephrotoxin.
   d. Possibility of toxic effects not affected by alcohol intake.
   e. Liver complications following exposure are rare.

219. The following are true regarding tetrachloroethane:
   a. Is a prescribed disease in cases of poisoning.
   b. Widely used as a general purpose solvent.
   c. Poisoning is associated with a toxic polyneuropathy.
   d. A renal syndrome is recognized as a feature of chronic exposure.
   e. Has proven teratogenic effects.

220. With regard to tetrachloroethylene (perchloroethylene) the following are correct:
   a. Widely used as a dry-cleaning fluid and decreasing agent.
   b. Not absorbed through the skin.
   c. Principal effect is CNS depression.
   d. Gamma-GT (gamma-glutamyltransferase) could be used in medical surveillance.
   e. Carcinogenic in workers chronically exposed.

221. In relation to methyl bromide the following are true:
   a. Is generally a colourless, odourless liquid which has a sweet smell in high concentration.
   b. Acute exposure may be associated with convulsions.
   c. Poisoning is a prescribed disease.
   d. Chronic exposure may lead to hepatic failure principally.
   e. Get a dry scaly rash in excessive skin exposure.

218. a. True
b. False Is lipid soluble and hence penetrates the skin.
c. True   Principally affecting the proximal tubules.
d. False High alcohol intake has a synergistic effect on carbon tetrachloride exposure.
e. False Is hepatotoxic. Get fatty degeneration and centrilobular necrosis.

219. a. True
b. False Rarely used. Has been replaced by other solvents due to its great toxicity.
c. True
d. False A hepatic syndrome which may lead to toxic jaundice and death has been described.
e. False

220. a. True   Has replaced trichloroethylene in this respect.
b. False Skin absorption is however limited. Inhalation is the main route of entry.
c. True   Causing narcotic effects.
d. True   Get elevated levels in exposed workers but account needs to be taken of other causes of elevated gamma-GT such as alcohol intake and liver disease.
e. False Although some studies in dry-cleaning industry have shown that it may be 'possibly carcinogenic in humans', carcinogenicity has not been fully established.

221. a. False It has these properties but is generally in gaseous form except at low temperatures (less than 4.5°C).
b. True   Is a very toxic gas. The convulsions may be difficult to control.
c. True
d. False May lead principally to renal failure. Also associated with peripheral neuropathy, optic atrophy and psychosis. Degenerative changes can however be seen in the liver.
e. False Get a characteristic erythematous, vesicular rash.

General toxicology

222. 111 – Trichloroethane (methyl chloroform) is:
   a. Commonly known as 'trike'.
   b. Being phased out of use in industry.
   c. Widely used for degreasing of metals.
   d. Teratogenic.
   e. Associated with fatalities.

223. Trichloroethylene:
   a. Is very volatile and rapidly absorbed through the lungs.
   b. Can cause peripheral nerve damage.
   c. Is associated with degreasers' flush.
   d. Is a severe skin irritant.
   e. May be a cause of sudden death due to ventricular fibrillation in young adults.

224. The following statements relating to solvent neurotoxicity are correct:
   a. Is related to lipid solubility.
   b. Carbon disulphide can cause Parkinsonism type symptoms.
   c. Pre-senile dementia is a feature of styrene poisoning.
   d. Addiction to solvents is a possibility.
   e. The neurotoxic effects are largely reversible.

225. With regard to vinyl chloride the following are true:
   a. Is a colourless gas used in the synthesis of polyvinyl chloride (PVC).
   b. Does not penetrate the skin.
   c. Is associated with scleroderma-like skin changes.
   d. Acro-osteolysis at distal ends of long bones is sometimes found in workers chronically exposed.
   e. Angiosarcoma of liver can be a feature of chronic poisoning.

226. In relation to nickel carbonyl the following are correct:
   a. Is formed in the Mond process.
   b. Is a highly toxic, colourless vapour rapidly absorbed via the lungs.
   c. In chronic poisoning raised levels of methaemoglobin are found.
   d. Poisoning is a prescribed industrial disease.
   e. Repeated exposure is associated with lung cancer.

General toxicology

222. a. False Trichloroethylene is known as 'trike'.
  b. True Under the *Montreal Protocol* its use is to be phased out by 1996.
  c. True Readily absorbed through the lungs and to a lesser extent via the skin. A mild irritant dermatitis may occur from skin contact.
  d. False Tests on experimental animals have not shown this.
  e. True Usually in cases of high exposure in confined spaces. In high concentrations get narcotic effects.

223. a. True
  b. False Can cause cranial nerve damage.
  c. True A facial vasodilatation in response to drinking alcohol.
  d. False A mild skin irritant.
  e. True Ventricular fibrillation can be induced by exertion following exposure.

224. a. True Lipid soluble substances can cross the blood–brain barrier and accumulate in nervous tissue.
  b. True As well as mixed polyneuropathies.
  c. False Associated with white spirit.
  d. True
  e. False

225. a. True
  b. False Can penetrate the skin but is rapidly absorbed through the lungs.
  c. True Affecting hands and forearms.
  d. False It affects the distal phalanges of the hands. Can cause a 'pseudoclubbing'.
  e. True Rare and confined to workers with extremely high exposures.

226. a. True
  b. True
  c. False May have raised levels of carboxyhaemoglobin due to associated carbon monoxide poisoning from the Mond process.
  d. True
  e. False Chronic exposure may lead to occupational asthma.

General toxicology

227. The following are correct with regard to hydrogen cyanide:
   a. The toxicity resides in the cyanide radicle.
   b. In poisoning cytochrome oxidase is blocked and hence oxygen transport.
   c. Symptoms of poisoning are of rapid onset and can be fatal.
   d. Treatment can involve the use of oxygen and amylnitrile capsules.
   e. Lactic acidosis is a prominent feature of poisoning.

228. With regard to pesticides the following are true:
   a. Poisoning with pesticides is not covered by *RIDDOR*.
   b. Neurotoxicity is a feature of many insecticides.
   c. Organochlorines persist in the environment for short periods.
   d. Organophosphate and carbamate groups inhibit acetylcholinesterase.
   e. The herbicide paraquat primarily affects the lungs.

General toxicology

227. a. True
b. False — Cytochrome oxidase is blocked which then interferes with oxygenation of tissues but oxygen transport is not affected.
c. True — Also headache, vomiting, excitability, convulsions.
d. True
e. True

228. a. False — They are reportable under *RIDDOR*.
b. True — By interfering with nerve impulse transmission.
c. False — Examples are DDT, Lindane. They last a long time in the environment.
d. True — Respiratory paralysis is the most serious and potentially fatal consequence of poisoning by organophosphates.
e. True — Rapidly absorbed by ingestion and specifically accumulates in lung tissue causing severe progressive lung damage. Liver damage and renal failure may also occur with poisoning.

Epidemiology and statistics

229. Epidemiology:
   a. Involves the study of the causes and distribution of disease in populations.
   b. Is partially useful in studying exposures at work.
   c. Uses a target population to infer to a study population.
   d. Utilizes sample populations when study populations are too large.
   e. Relies on tests of statistical significance as the basis on which all investigations are performed.

Match the following:

230. Sensitivity.
231. Specificity.
232. Efficiency.
233. Validity.
234. Repeatability.

   a. Representing a true assessment of what it measures and compares with established methods.
   b. Detection of a high proportion of true positives.
   c. An expression of the extent of agreement between repeated measurements in the same subject under same conditions.
   d. Related to the proportion of all subjects tested who have been correctly diagnosed or classified.
   e. Detection of a high proportion of false negatives which are classified as negative by a test.

235. The following statements are correct with regard to screening tests:
   a. Must be sensitive and specific.
   b. Involve conditions with a recognizable latent or early symptomatic stage.
   c. Are useful in developing new treatment regimes.
   d. Predictive value is linked to disease incidence.
   e. Are cross-sectional in nature.

229. a. True
 b. False Is very useful in studying how workplace exposures and practices influence the health of persons at work.
 c. False Uses a study population from which it is hoped to infer to a target population.
 d. True
 e. False Results of some epidemiological investigation may be purely descriptive in content.

230. b. High sensitivity implies a low false negative rate.

231. e. A test is specific if there are few false positives.

232. d. This is a measure of the overall success of a test in correctly classifying subjects.

233. a.

234. c. Also known as 'reproducibility'.

235. a. True
 b. True Facilities must also exist for diagnosis and treatment.
 c. False Accepted treatment regimes should be in place prior to introducing a screening test.
 d. False It is linked to prevalence – the higher the prevalence of a condition the better the predictive value of the screening test.
 e. True Involves surveying a population at a point in time to detect early disease amenable to treatment.

Epidemiology and statistics

236. In relation to standardized mortality ratio (SMR) the following are correct:
   a. Can be used to compare mortality risk between different occupations.
   b. A value of less than 100 indicates a higher than expected mortality experience.
   c. Takes account of social class.
   d. Affected by the 'healthy worker effect'.
   e. Unaffected by the 'survivor effect'.

Match the following:

237. Prevalence rate.
238. Incidence rate.
239. Standardized mortality ratio.
240. Odds ratio.
241. Proportional mortality ratio.

a. The number of a population at risk who develop a condition within a stated time period.
b. A weighted average of the ratios of age-specific mortality proportions in two groups.
c. A measure of the risk of disease in a study population compared to that of a reference population.
d. The number of a population who have a condition at a given time or over a stated period of time.
e. An age-standardized measure of mortality in a study group relative to that in a reference group.

242. The following are true with regard to a cohort study:
   a. A prospective study of a group of people defined by some common aspect of their occupational history.
   b. Small numbers are sufficient.
   c. An example of a longitudinal study.
   d. Suitable for exploring new hypotheses.
   e. May be expensive and time consuming.

236. a. True Listed in Registrar General's 'Occupational Mortality Tables'.
b. False Values above 100 indicate this. Values for SMR that are less than 100 indicate a lower than expected mortality experience.
c. False SMR does not take account of social class differences. Thus the mortality effects due to occupation must be separated out from those due to social class, e.g. by using wives as a social class control group.
d. True Certain occupations require a high standard of fitness and hence that occupation selects 'fitter subjects' which is reflected in the SMR (healthy worker effect).
e. False Certain occupations have a high fitness standard which forces those with illness to leave. Thus those left in such an occupation tend to be fitter ('survivor effect'). This selection effect makes SMR prone to bias.

237. d. This is point prevalence and period prevalence. Prevalence rates are affected by the prognosis of a medical condition.

238. a. Refers to new cases only. Not affected by prognosis of a medical condition.

239. e. SMR is $(O/E \times 100)$ where O = number of observed deaths in a study population and E = the expected number of deaths. A value for an SMR greater than 100 indicates a higher number of deaths in the study group than expected.

240. c.

241. b. This measures the proportion of deaths in a cohort group and compares it to the proportion of deaths in the general population. A figure greater than 100 indicates a higher proportion of deaths in the cohort group.

242. a. True
b. False Tend to involve large numbers.
c. True
d. False Not suitable as they can only be undertaken where evidence already exists for cause and effect.
e. True

Epidemiology and statistics

243. In relation to a case control study the following are true:
a. Need larger numbers than a cohort study.
b. Should be at least twice as many cases as controls.
c. Cases and controls should be matched for confounding variables.
d. Not susceptible to selection bias.
e. An example of a retrospective study.

244. With regard to cross-sectional studies the following are true:
a. Capable of giving dynamic pictures.
b. Essentially studies of survivors.
c. Easy and quick to complete.
d. May not involve any statistical inference.
e. Study population may be atypical with reference to target population.

Match the following:

245. Mean.

246. Mode.

247. Median.

248. Frequency distribution curve.

249. Normal distribution curve.

a. The value of a variable which has the highest frequency.
b. The sum of all observed values divided by the number of observations.
c. Shows the underlying distribution of a variable in an infinitely large population.
d. Is unimodal, bell-shaped and completely symmetrical about its mean.
e. The middle value of a series of observations placed in either ascending or descending order.

243. a. False   Usually needs fewer numbers than cohort study.
    b. False   Should be more controls than cases with the ideal ratio around 4:1.
    c. True   Confounding variables include age, sex, smoking, etc.
    d. False   Bias may occur in selection of both cases and controls.
    e. True   Is a comparison between a group with a disease (cases) and a group without (controls) with respect to their past exposure to possible risk factors for that disease.

244. a. False   Provide only a snapshot or static picture of the study population.
    b. True   No account is taken of deaths, retirements or sickness absence.
    c. True
    d. True
    e. True

245. b. The value of the mean can be influenced by a few isolated high or low values ('outliers').

246. a. Not widely used as may get a spurious result when the number of observations is small.

247. e. Not affected by outliers.

248. c.

249. d. Also known as a 'Gaussian distribution'. Here the value of the mean, mode and median is the same.

Epidemiology and statistics

250. The following are true regarding audit:
a. Does not apply to occupational health and safety.
b. Legislation implies audit should take place.
c. Is an expensive process for industry with no return.
d. Can involve measuring performance and setting targets.
e. Can help to ensure a safer working environment for employees.

Match the following:

251. Standard deviation.	a.	The variability of sample means in relation to the population value.
252. Standard error.	b.	Indicates the relationship between one set of variables and another using the slope of a line drawn to represent them.
253. Correlation coefficient.		
254. Confidence intervals.	c.	A range of values within which a particular statistic value lies.
255. Regression coefficient.	d.	A measure of the dispersion of values about their mean.
	e.	Measures the strength of a linear relationship between two variables.

256. With regard to statistical tests the following are correct:
a. Help decide if the difference between two sample statistics are due to sample variation or if they are in reality different.
b. Usually used to test the null hypothesis.
c. Statistical significance can be equated with clinical significance.
d. Samples used need not be random.
e. Chi-squared test compares sample proportions.

Epidemiology and statistics

250.
- a. False — Audit can assess the processes or their outcomes involved in all areas of occupational health and safety.
- b. True — HSAWA and the *Management Regulations* imply that health and safety measures should be subject to audit.
- c. False — May contribute to reducing costs due to accidents and ill health. May also identify areas to improve production.
- d. True — Audit is a cyclical process involving the straightforward objective comparison of aspects of performance with agreed standards set as targets.
- e. True — Within the bounds of practicability.

251. d. One of the most widely used measures of variation. A low standard deviation implies high reproducibility.

252. a. A large value indicates the means are widely dispersed about the population mean.

253. e. The value ranges from +1 to −1. If it is positive this indicates both variables increase together.

254. c. Expressed as either 99 per cent or 95 per cent confidence intervals.

255. b.

256.
- a. True — In other words are the differences due to chance or are they due to some inter-relation or other variant.
- b. True — Start off with the premise that there is no difference between study groups.
- c. False — A statistically significant result in a study may have no clinical (practical) importance.
- d. False — When sampling for the purposes of these tests the method used must ensure randomization of selection.
- e. True — Chi-squared test is used to gain a measure of the overall difference between observed and expected measurements.

Appendix A: Common causes of occupational asthma

Chemical

Acid anhydrides (epoxy resin)
Aluminium
Amines (epoxy resin)
Chromates
Cobalt
Di-isocyanates
Formaldehyde
Glutaraldehyde
Perchlorates
Nickel
Platinum salts
Vanadium

Vegetable agents

Colophony (pine resin)
Mahogany
Western red cedar
Flour, grain

Microbiological

B. Subtilis enzymes (detergents)
Fungal antigens

Animals

Grain mites
Horses, dogs, cats
Insects
Rats and other rodents

Pharmaceuticals

Cephalosporins
Methyldopa
Penicillins

Appendix B: Common causes of occupational dermatitis

Allergic contact dermatitis

Nickel
Chrome salts (cement)
Rubber
Epoxy resin
Colophony
Cobalt
Formaldehyde
Glutaraldehyde
Dyes
Plants
Cosmetics
Antibiotics
Mercury
Hardwoods

Irritant contact dermatitis

Alkalis
Detergents
Solvents
Cutting oils
Cement
Fibreglass

Appendix C: Occupations associated with contact dermatitis

Engineering
Building, insulation and cement-casting
Cleaning
Hairdressing
Rubber and plastics
Woodworking
Hotel and restaurant
Hospital and laboratory
Floristry
Agriculture and horticulture
Painting
Adhesive and sealant
Lathe operators
Soldering

Appendix D: Occupational exposure limits

The table below gives some examples of occupational exposure limits. They are shown as long-term values, taken as an eight-hour time weighted average (TWA) or short-term exposure limits (STEL) of ten minutes.

COSHH Regulations recognize two types of occupational exposure limit (i) OES – occupational exposure standard and (ii) MEL – maximum exposure limit. Both are used to determine adequate control of exposure to a substance by inhalation.

Occupational exposure standard – the level of concentration of an airborne substance at which harmful side effects are unlikely to occur to an employee exposed by inhalation day in day out. It is averaged out over a reference period and takes account of current scientific knowledge. If the OES is not exceeded then exposure control is regarded as adequate.

Maximal exposure limit – the maximum level of concentration of an airborne substance to which employees may be exposed by inhalation under any circumstances. It is averaged over a reference period and all reasonable steps have to be taken to reduce exposures below the MEL as far as is reasonably practicable.

Lists of OESs and MELs are found in the Health and Safety Executive annually updated publication *EH40, Occupational Exposure Limits*. Further explanation of both limits are found in *EH40* and *EH64, Occupational Exposure Limits; Criteria Document Summaries*.

An additional feature in the table below is the notation used in *EH40*. This identifies those substances which exhibit significant skin absorption (skin) and those with respiratory sensitization properties (sensitizer).

Substance	Eight-hour TWA	Short term (10 min)	Notation
* Acetic anhydride		5 ppm	
* Acetone	750 ppm	1500 ppm	
** Acrylamide	0.3 mg.m^{-3}		Skin
** Acrylonitrile	2 ppm		Skin
* Aluminium metal	10 mg.m^{-3} (total inhalable dust)		

Appendix D: Occupational exposure limits

* Aluminium oxide	5 mg.m^{-3} (respirable dust) 10 mg.m^{-3} (total inhalable dust) 5 mg.m^{-3} (respirable dust)		
* Ammonia	25 ppm	35 ppm	
** Arsenic and compounds	0.1 mg.m^{-3}		
** Benzene	5 ppm		
** Bis (chloromethyl) ether (BCME)	0.001 ppm		
**Buta-1,3-diene	10 ppm		
* Butan-1-oL		50 ppm	Skin
** 2-Butoxyethanol	25 ppm		Skin
* n-Butylamine		5 ppm	Skin
** Carbon disulphide	10 ppm		Skin
* Carbon tetrachloride	2 ppm		Skin
* Chlorine	0.5 ppm	1 ppm	
* Chlorine trifluoride		0.1 ppm	
* Chloroacetaldehyde		1 ppm	
* Chlorobenzene	50 ppm		
* Chlorodifluoromethane	1000 ppm		
* 2-Chloroethanol		1 ppm	Skin
* Chloroform	2 ppm		Skin
** Chromium inorganic compounds	0.05 mg.m^{-3}		
* Copper fume	0.2 mg.m^{-3}		
* Cumene	25 ppm	75 ppm	
* Cyanogen chloride		0.3 ppm	
* Cyclohexane	100 ppm	300 ppm	
** 1,2-Dibromoethane	0.5 ppm		Skin
* Dichloroacetylene		0.1 ppm	
* 1,2-Dichlorobenzene		50 ppm	
* 1,4-Dichlorobenzene	25 ppm	50 ppm	
* 1,1-Dichloroethane	200 ppm	400 ppm	
** 2,2^1-Dichloro-4,4^1-methylene dianiline (MbOCA)	0.005 mg.m^{-3}		Skin
* N,N-Dimethylethylamine	10 ppm	15 ppm	
* Disulphur dichloride		1 ppm	
** 2-Ethoxyethanol	10 ppm		Skin
** 2-Ethoxyethyl acetate	10 ppm		Skin
** Ethylene oxide	5 ppm		
* Fluorine		1 ppm	
** Formaldehyde	2 ppm	2 ppm	
* Glutaraldehyde		0.2 ppm	
** Grain dust	10 mg.m^{-3}		

Appendix D: Occupational exposure limits

* n-Hexane	20 ppm		
* Hydrogen bromide		3 ppm	
* Hydrogen chloride		5 ppm	
** Hydrogen cyanide		10 ppm	Skin
* Hydrogen fluoride (as F)		3 ppm	
* Iodine		0.1 ppm	
** Isocyanates	0.02 mg.m^{-3}	0.07 mg.m^{-3}	Sensitizer
* Isopropyl acetate		200 ppm	
Lead and compounds (lead-in-air standard)	0.15 mg.m^{-3}		
* Lithium hydroxide (total inhalable dust)		1 mg.m^{-3}	
* Magnesium oxide (as Mg)	5 mg.m^{-3} (fume, respirable dust) 10 mg.m^{-3} (total inhalable dust)	10 mg.m^{-3} (fume respirable dust)	
* Manganese and compounds (dust)	5 mg.m^{-3}		
** Man-made mineral fibre	5 mg.m^{-3} (total inhalable dust) 2 fibres/ml (fibre count)		
** 2-Methoxyethanol	5 ppm		Skin
** 2-Methoxyethyl acetate	5 ppm		Skin
* Methyl acrylate	10 ppm		
* 1-Methylbutyl acetate		150 ppm	
* Monochloroacetic acid	0.3 ppm		Skin
** Nickel	0.5 mg.m^{-3}		
* 4-Nitroaniline	6 mg.m^{-3}		Skin
* 2,2-Oxydiethanol	100 mg.m^{-3}		
* 2-Phenylpropene		100 ppm	
* Phosphine		0.3 ppm	
* Piperidine	1 ppm		Skin
* Portland cement dust	10 mg.m^{-3} (total inhalable dust) 5 mg.m^{-3} (respirable dust)		
* Potassium hydroxide		2 mg.m^{-3}	
* Propane-1,2-diol	150 ppm (vapour and particulate)		
** Rubber fume	0.6 mg.m^{-3}		

Appendix D: Occupational exposure limits

* Selenium and compounds	0.1 mg.m^{-3}		
** Silica (respirable crystalline dust)	0.4 mg.m^{-3}		
* Silver compounds	0.01 mg.m^{-3}		
* Sodium hydroxide		2 mg.m^{-3}	
** Styrene	100 ppm	250 ppm	
* Terphenyls		0.5 ppm	
* Tetrachloroethylene	50 ppm	150 ppm	
Tetraethyl lead (lead-in-air standard)	0.10 mg.m^{-3}		
* Toluene	50 ppm	150 ppm	Skin
** 1,1,1-Trichloroethane	350 ppm	450 ppm	
** Trichloroethylene	100 ppm	150 ppm	Skin
* Trinitrotoluene	0.5 mg.m^{-3}		Skin
** Vinyl chloride	7 ppm		
** Vinylidene chloride	10 ppm		
** Wood dust (hardwood) (total inhalable dust)	5 mg.m^{-3}		Sensitizer
* Xylene	100 ppm	150 ppm	Skin

* = OES
** = MEL

Further reading

Recommended texts – general references

Edwards, F.C., McCallum, R.I. and Taylor, P.J. (eds), *Fitness For Work – The Medical Aspects.* Oxford Medical Publications (1994)
Farmer, R. and Miller D., *Lecture Notes on Epidemiology and Public Health.* 3rd edition. Blackwell Science (1991)
Harrington, J.M. and Gill, F.S., *Occupational Health.* 3rd edition. Blackwell Scientific (1992)
Raffle, P.A.B., Adams, P., Baxter, P.S. and Lee, W.R. (eds), *Hunter's Diseases of Occupation.* 8th edition. Edward Arnold (1994)
Rom, W.N. (ed), *Environmental and Occupational Medicine.* Little, Brown & Co (1992)
Seaton, A., Agius, R., McCloy, E. and D'Auria, D. *Practical Occupational Medicine.* 1st edition. Edward Arnold (1994)
Waldron, H.A., *Occupational Health Practice.* 3rd edition. Butterworth-Heinemann (1989)
Waldron, H.A., *Lecture Notes on Occupational Medicine.* 4th edition. Blackwell Scientific (1990).

Specialist texts

Ashton, I. and Gill, I.S. *Monitoring for Health Hazards at Work.* Blackwell Scientific (1992)
Clayton, G.D. and Clayton, F.E. (eds). *Pattys Industrial Hygiene and Toxicology.* 4th edition. John Wiley and Sons (1991).
Griffiths, W.A.D. and Wilkinson, D.S. (eds). *Essentials of Industrial Dermatology.* Blackwell Scientific (1985)
Parkes, W.R. *Occupational Lung Disorders.* 3rd edition. Butterworth-Heinemann (1994)

Journals

Occupational and Environmental Medicine.
Journal of Occupational Medicine.
Occupational Health.
Occupational Health Review.

Useful addresses

Faculty of Occupational Medicine
Royal College of Physicians
6 St Andrews Place
Regents Park
London NW1 4LE

Faculty of Occupational Medicine
Royal College of Physicians of Ireland
6 Kildare Street
Dublin 2

Society of Occupational Medicine
6 St Andrews Place
Regents Park
London NW1 4LE

Royal College of Nursing Society of Occupational Health Nursing
20 Cavendish Square
London W1M OAB

Health and Safety Executive Information Centre
Broad Lane
Sheffield S3 7HQ

Health and Safety Agency for Northern Ireland
83 Ladas Drive
Belfast BT6 9FJ

Printed in the United Kingdom
by Lightning Source UK Ltd.
120161UK00001B/23